'Nick Pole has performed a real service by showing how Clean Language is something everyone can use. It is a pleasure to see my late friend David Grove's work receiving such practical explication and application. This is a how-to manual suitable for anyone who wants to be better at working with the wisdom within each of us.'
– *Ian McDermott, Founder of International Teaching Seminars and UKCP-certified psychotherapist*

'Nick Pole has written an important and convincing book. Spoken language and body language have drifted apart. *Words that Touch* introduces how to make dialogue an integral part of bodywork. Without any doubt many therapists and teachers of bodywork will find inspiration and practical guidance in it.'
– *Peter den Dekker, Chi Kung instructor, acupuncturist and author of* The Dynamics of Standing Still

'*Words that Touch* gently balances the Ying and Yang of language and body, theory and practice with hundreds of stories, examples and personal anecdotes. Nick Pole's delightful book shows how Clean Language questions can transcend technique to become a way of being with another person's body and mind.'
– *James Lawley and Penny Tompkins, authors of* Metaphors in Mind: Transformation through Symbolic Modelling

WORDS
that Touch

of related interest

SEI-KI
Life in Resonance – The Secret Art of Shiatsu
Akinobu Kishi and Alice Whieldon
ISBN 978 1 84819 042 9
eISBN 978 0 85701 260 9

EVERY BODY TELLS A STORY
A Craniosacral Journey
Liz Kalinowska and Daška Hatton
ISBN 978 1 84819 268 3
eISBN 978 1 78450 281 2

MIND CLEARING
The Key to Mindfulness Mastery
Alice Whieldon
Foreword by Lawrence Noyes
ISBN 978 1 84905 307 5
eISBN 978 0 85700 637 0

AWAKENING SOMATIC INTELLIGENCE
Understanding, Learning & Practicing the Alexander
Technique, Feldenkrais Method & Hatha Yoga
Graeme Lynn
ISBN 978 1 84819 334 5
eISBN 978 0 85701 290 6

WORDS
that Touch

How to Ask Questions
Your Body Can Answer

12 ESSENTIAL 'CLEAN QUESTIONS' FOR MIND/BODY THERAPISTS

NICK POLE

ILLUSTRATIONS BY SOPHIE STANDING

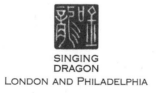

SINGING
DRAGON
LONDON AND PHILADELPHIA

First published in 2017
by Singing Dragon
an imprint of Jessica Kingsley Publishers
73 Collier Street
London N1 9BE, UK
and
400 Market Street, Suite 400
Philadelphia, PA 19106, USA

www.singingdragon.com

Library of Congress Cataloging in Publication Data
A CIP catalog record for this book is available from the Library of Congress

British Library Cataloguing in Publication Data
A CIP catalogue record for this book is available from the British Library

ISBN 978 1 84819 336 9
eISBN 978 0 85701 292 0

Printed and bound in Great Britain

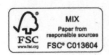

To the memory of my dad, historian Jack Pole,
who liked to quote Ecclesiastes 12:12:

'...*by these, my son, be admonished: of making many books
there is no end, and much study is a weariness of the flesh.*'

CONTENTS

ACKNOWLEDGEMENTS

How do you thank everyone who has helped you to create a book? On one hand, it is a wonderful exercise in the clinically proven benefits of feeling and expressing gratitude. On the other, you risk the embarrassingly effusive tone of an over-long Oscar acceptance speech. So let me keep this short and thank all those who gave me their critical comments and enthusiastic encouragement, usually in equal measure, and all those members of the Clean community who generously agreed to be interviewed. To preserve confidentiality, many who I need to thank are not mentioned by name, but you know who you are. Those who I can publicly acknowledge, and who in one way or another, directly or indirectly, have given me the inspiration, encouragement or support that I needed to make this book a reality, are, in alphabetical order:

Alice Whieldon

Ann Weiser Cornell

Bill O'Hanlon

Bill Palmer

Caitlin Walker

Carola Beresford-Cooke

Gary Born

Ian McDermott

James Lawley

Jessica Kingsley

Katerina Pylava

Michael Lomvardos

Michael Mallows

Penny Tompkins

Peter den Dekker

Philipp Walz

Rachel Henke

Rogan Wolf

Stephen Porges

Steve Gilligan

Suzi Caunce

Tomas Nelissen

Verena Schwalm

Wendy Sullivan

Wolfgang Löffler

Many thanks also to all my colleagues in the UK Shiatsu College, and, of course, my wife Katharine, who reminded me that the Clean approach is not always the best when, after I had already been working on this project for far too long, gave me the best advice any writer could ever hope for: 'Just finish the f*cking book!'

HOMECOMING

It's as if the landscape

gathers you into its arms

and makes you

not just welcome here

but whole.

It has reached out and found

you where you alone

could not. You are never lost

among these contours.

They map your interior.

You are discovered here.

Rogan Wolf

PART 1
THE BASICS

~ 1 ~

A LONG WAY FROM YOURSELF

My Japanese shiatsu teacher never said much when I went to see him for a treatment. He would simply give me a cheerful smile and wave at the mat. The message could not have been clearer: 'Words are not important here.' What he did, how he listened, inquired, suggested or questioned, he did in silence. The qualities of his presence, warmth and total attention made a session with him seem more like a tea ceremony performed through touch than the normal mixture of detailed questioning and advice-giving I was used to in most forms of bodywork. Sometimes at the end he would smile again and ask, 'Did you enjoy the treatment?' I never knew what to say to that, since entertainment wasn't what I thought I'd come for, and anyway, it seemed like his way of discouraging any attempt to think about or analyse what had happened in the session.

Then one evening, my treatment was the last one of his long day and afterwards he invited me to sit down with him while he relaxed. He poured me a glass of wine, and one for himself, and after a bit of talk of other things, fixed me with a friendly but frighteningly penetrating gaze and said, 'You are a long way from yourself.' It took me by surprise; I felt confused. I probably nodded; perhaps I managed a wry smile and pretended to know exactly what he meant. I do remember a defiant little voice inside me wanting to say, 'That's what you think!' Even then I was a keen student of how language can be integrated with bodywork to help the client make some sense of what they experience in a session, and the words he'd offered me broke all the rules. They weren't framed as a question, they had no relation to anything I'd said to him, they were his opinion, not mine, and they certainly invited no reply. At least, I couldn't think of one at the time.

At another level, of course, he was absolutely right. It took me maybe 15 years to find the self that he was talking about, the self that cared enough about the possibilities of integrating language with bodywork to eventually get this book into your hands. But I still wonder what might have happened if, instead of just leaving me with a koan, a conundrum, he had asked me a few simple questions, with that same gentle, compassionate, demanding curiosity his hands conveyed through touch – a few simple questions that might have given my stubborn mind some sense of the self I was so far away from.

When I first discovered Clean Language, I was struck by the way it seemed to do with words what he could do with touch. There is something very Japanese, very Zen, about it, about the way, by using the fewest and simplest words, it can create the potential for profound change. Clients not only experience real insights, they also feel the somatic shifts that show that insight has been embodied and embedded. And there is the same deep respect for empty space, a listening clarity that doesn't interfere, which simply waits to be met. My teacher's way of working with the body was usually very gentle but it could also sometimes be energetic, emphatic – more Aikido then tea ceremony – but it never seemed imposed on you. It came from a simple willingness to sit, to respect the other person's space, to leave a kind of a stillness in which the slightest ripple might be the start of a whole process. Clean Language seemed to mirror all this by keeping formal structure and technique to an absolute minimum. In fact, it seemed the perfect complement to my teacher's way of working with the body, since both methods seemed to allow as pure as possible a response to what was really coming from the client.

VERBAL MIND AND BODYMIND

When I started to integrate Clean Language with bodywork, this opened up a very special possibility. Any bodywork therapist knows how hard it is to describe in words what we actually do: what it's really like to engage with another person's physical being and perhaps all the rest of their being, with movement or touch. And for most of our clients too it's just as challenging to find words for their experience of that. One reason for this is that the parts of the brain that are most directly involved in processing language do not find it easy to communicate with the parts of the brain that give us our somatic sense of self. Both sides of the brain are involved in each of these functions, of course, but there is a growing consensus among neuroscientists interested in mindfulness and the mind/body connection that what I will call the 'verbal mind' lives mostly in the left hemisphere, while the right hemisphere has much more direct access to that somatic sense of self which I will call the 'bodymind'. Though I can only put this in a very simplified way (and one that would make any self-respecting neuroscientist cringe), research that you can read more about in Part 2 suggests these two kinds of mind communicate in very different ways and have very different priorities. As far as the verbal mind is concerned, feelings don't really exist until they have a name, some kind of label by which they can be recognised and fitted into an existing structure. But for the bodymind, those labels can often seem like an attempt to close down any real dialogue between conceptual knowledge and felt experience. To call a knee pain 'arthritis', or a chronic gut problem 'irritable bowel', may be medically accurate but doesn't help the client to connect with their knee or their gut in any healing way; in fact it tends to cut off communication with the symptoms and sensations which are the native language of the body.

When we ask 'Clean' questions, the opposite happens. By focusing attention on a symptom, and by asking the kind of questions that we do, the body begins to sense that it is being listened to in an entirely different way, perhaps in a way that it has never experienced before. Because Clean questions make no judgements and bring an absolute minimum of presupposition to the dialogue, they leave room for all the subtlety and ambiguity which is a natural part of how our bodies process information and communicate. The normally dominant verbal mind, with its tendency to think of the body simply as a machine made up of individual parts, can easily become impatient with this. It prefers to use language as a way to categorise than to connect, language that takes the client away from their direct experience of the body. Clean Language, on the other hand, brings the spotlight of attention to the very simplest elements of experience, the ones that are hidden most of the time by the artificial complexities that the verbal mind is constantly trying to create.

Using words in this way offers me a way to interact with my clients at almost the same level as I would by using touch. At the same time, it involves the client in the process and brings their body into the conversation as an equal partner. This means that when we arrive at a point where the client feels ready to begin the bodywork, there is already a triangle of trust between their verbal mind, their bodymind and me. For me as the practitioner, that trust gives the work a truly enjoyable depth and flow, a flow that comes from somewhere my verbal mind has almost no connection with.

Clients often say, after any kind of bodywork, how much more in touch they feel with themselves. That's not surprising, because no matter how much the verbal mind likes to deny it, a genuine sense of self is always a meeting between body and mind. As bodywork therapists, we are expert at working with the body but rarely get specific training in how to work with our client's verbal mind. Clean Language is an elegant way to bridge that gap.

These simple questions give the verbal mind the tools it needs to begin a dialogue with the body: a dialogue which most of our clients will never have thought was possible before.

∽ 2 ∽

WHY CLEAN LANGUAGE?

This book is intended as a friendly and practical guide to using Clean Language in bodywork therapy. How you define bodywork is up to you. You may be a physiotherapist, CranioSacral therapist or shiatsu practitioner, for example, and want to help your clients connect with their own inner responses as they learn to inhabit their bodies in new ways. Maybe you're an acupuncturist wanting to make sense of the peculiar metaphors your clients come up with under the influence of your strategically placed needles; perhaps you teach yoga or qi gong or Feldenkrais and are looking for ways for your clients to give language to movement; you may even be a mindfulness teacher, or a psychotherapist working mainly with words but curious about how people can connect more easily with bodily sensations and the meanings behind them. In all of these, Clean Language offers enormous potential for helping clients make their own sense of what is going on for them, both in the treatment room and as they take your work with them back into their everyday lives.

Clean Language is now being used in areas like education, business, medicine and government as well as in the world of therapy where it began. Its simplicity, accessibility and adaptability help to explain that growing popularity. When someone asks you Clean questions in a skilful way, you can't help but notice that those questions seem to come from a place of profound respect for, and curiosity about, you and your relationship with yourself, and that they offer a surprisingly direct way to the heart of any problem that's affecting that relationship. Clean questions help us realise we know more about ourselves than we thought we knew. In fact they can take us to the edge of what we can say with words and sometimes beyond that, inviting us to step into wordless space where we may fall like Alice down our own personal rabbit holes; or fly through, above or beyond the landscapes of our everyday sense of the mind/body relationship, seeing familiar obstacles from a new perspective and making new connections between different parts of that landscape – all because someone knew how to ask us the right kind of question, in the right way, at the right moment.

In bodywork therapy, Clean questions give the conscious mind a better sense of just how intimately it is connected to the body, and they give the body a chance to express itself in ways the mind can understand. When you work with the body, Clean questions focus the mind in a constructive way on the meaning of physical symptoms, and when the mind starts listening to the body then the body begins to respond. Physical pain usually becomes less intense, stuck feelings begin to shift and the somatic self begins to communicate through images, emotions, memories and metaphors rather than simply through pain. And as the verbal mind learns to listen to this other side of itself, the body begins to have more trust in it. Clients discover that parts of themselves that they felt cut off from, angry with or fearful of, may actually have vital clues to offer to the verbal mind, with its unique abilities to organise, plan and make things happen, as it picks its way along the path towards living a more embodied life.

Clean Language is also about listening to words not just as labels for things – cognitive playing cards that we shuffle around in our heads – but as things in themselves, whose sounds and rhythms and the way they are spoken can have their own meaning. It's about how to listen to a word or phrase or gesture that someone offers you and get the best sense you can of what resonances it has for that person, before offering it back to them in the form of a beautifully simple and functional question. If we are interested in helping our clients listen more effectively to themselves, Clean questions are especially useful because they lead our attention away from a mainly verbal understanding, through all the neurological activity that makes up a thought, via the nerves, muscle trains, connective tissue and energy channels, to the embodied sense of what these particular words or gestures really mean to that person, and why it matters that they should have uttered them just now. When someone asks me a Clean question in this way, I'm immediately aware of something different going on; it's as though the question has come from somewhere beyond any roles we might be playing with each other and beyond any theories about how therapy should work.

This is because, compared to most traditional bodywork therapies, Clean Language takes a fundamentally different approach to what needs to happen between client and practitioner. There are literally hundreds of schools of bodywork therapy, and like schools of fish, they swim mostly in the same sea, one where it is presupposed that a well-tempered and skilful practitioner in some way guides the client's self-healing process via the theories, values, metaphors and diagnostic frameworks of whatever therapy they are trained in. Even though a lot may be said nowadays about empowering the client and building a therapeutic partnership, in most complementary therapies the practitioner's job is to diagnose what is wrong with the client and do what's necessary to put it right, just as it is in conventional medical care; the client does not need to understand or even believe in how the therapy works; all they need to do is patiently receive the treatment until it restores them to health. There's nothing wrong with that model: it's one that we all need sometimes, and it remains the one that most people expect when they come to us for help. But over the past 50 years, a different approach to what happens between client and therapist has been evolving, and new ways to use language to facilitate mind/body communication (which mostly have their roots in Gestalt or Eugene Gendlin's Focusing, or both) have emerged.

Clean Language is one of these – a particularly simple one – which offers you ways to help clients become more self-aware, take more responsibility and do more of the work in a session, and to learn more about themselves in the process. Of course, for many if not most of our clients, this may be the last thing they want to do. But if you have ever spent time as a patient in the normal medical system, being moved from one expert to another and one department to another (undergoing strange and invasive tests and procedures), or if you've ever experienced any kind of bodywork therapy without understanding the first thing about how it actually works, it can be very liberating to discover that such simple questions can open you up to yourself in such a direct and enlightening way.

This book is not intended to turn your work as a mind/body practitioner into some kind of amateur psychotherapy. What it will do is make it easier for your clients to be clear about what they want, to be more aware of and curious about shifts that happen in the treatment, to learn an exceptionally effective way of being more attentive to themselves and their symptoms, and to take more responsibility for putting all of this into practice in their daily lives. Clean Language seems to resonate perfectly with the quality of attention that is such a fundamental part of many healing traditions. At the same time, it helps you to clarify and respect your own boundaries as well your client's. In doing so it creates an extraordinary space between the two of you, one whose very emptiness seems paradoxically to nourish all those qualities of presence, empathy, compassion and courage that every therapist, and every client, needs. If that sounds like something you have been looking for, then let me welcome you to the world of Clean and begin to explain just what it's all about.

~ 3 ~

KEEPING IT CLEAN AND
WHY IT MATTERS

When you use Clean questions in bodywork therapy, you're working at the delicate interface between mind and muscle, between thought, sensation, emotion and impulse. To experience this, just take a moment to clear your head, take a breath or two, reconnect with your sense of how your body feels right now, and then notice as sensitively as you can, in both mind and body, what happens when you try to answer each of the following questions:

1. What is an equilateral triangle?

2. How does your lower back feel right now?

3. Can you think of a place where you'd love to be?

What happened? You probably noticed a different sort of mind/body experience depending on whether you were being asked a mental kind of question (the first one), a physical one (the second) or an emotional or even spiritual one (the third). And notice how, to answer the first one, you probably went somewhere inside your head; to answer the second one your attention had to go to your lower back; and to answer the third one you probably had to go outside yourself in some way.

Every time you ask someone a question, you're directing – in a sense manipulating – their focus of attention. Most of the time we do this completely unconsciously, but when you learn how to ask Clean questions, you immediately notice how the questions themselves filter out your normal conversational or diagnostic impulses. When those are gone, the space between client and practitioner becomes unusually clear – and that clarity leaves the person answering the questions free to explore another kind of space, their own inner space, putting into words the sensations, emotions, movements and resonances that are a direct expression of the very patterns we want to work with as bodywork therapists.

DEFINING 'CLEAN'

So why is it called 'Clean' Language? This is important. Some therapists take offence at the implication that if the language they use with their clients isn't 'Clean' then it must somehow be 'dirty'. The name may be provocative, but the aim behind it is to be as respectful as possible to your client's subjective reality, in all its subtlety, depth and complexity. So if you want a definition of Clean Language, I would say:

> *Clean Language is a set of questions that help the client to explore and transform their own subjective reality with minimum interference from the questioner.*

Like most definitions, it raises a few questions. The thing Clean Language is best known for is its claim to keep the client's space as clear as possible of any subjective influence from whoever is asking the questions. The aim is to create a form of dialogue that naturally filters out the kind of conversational clutter that normal conversations, including many therapeutic ones, usually contain. Asking Clean questions is like learning another language. Until you are fluent, the mind can get very busy planning what to say next.

On top of that, it often starts to worry about saying the wrong thing, or how the client will react. As the practitioner, it sounds strange to repeat back the client's words so exactly; won't it sound strange? Won't they just get irritated with all these questions and want to get on with the treatment? And on top of that, of course, the habits of normal conversation keep popping into your head – all the other things you would usually say instead of Clean questions, all the things you usually rely on because you know they work. As you read through this list of the tactics we unthinkingly employ in everyday conversation, you may remember something a therapist once said to you that just didn't 'fit' for you, or maybe sounded more like what they wanted to say than what you meant them to hear:

Preconceptions: for example, about how therapy should work, or about what your weight should be.

Judgements: 'Why is he avoiding the issue?' or 'Why is she wearing those shoes with that top?'

Prejudices: usually these are either unconscious or zealously suppressed, especially around issues like race, class, gender, sexual orientation, social status or financial wealth, but Clean questions make them easier to notice.

Opinions: 'I'm not sure your therapist is really helping you.'

Advice: 'You just need to let it go.'

Analysis: 'Your mother's pain is at the root of this.'

Mind reading: 'I know just how you feel.'

Interpretations: 'All this neck tension is a sign of family trauma.'

Stories: 'The exact same thing happened to me once...'

Diagnosis: in all the subtle ways it can infiltrate your way of being present with your client.

Non-verbal comments: for example, the expression on your face when the client says something you don't agree with.

In other words, everything that the busy minds of both client and practitioner might want to fill that empty space with. When you start learning how to ask Clean questions, it sometimes feels that so much of your normal way of carrying on a conversation has been stripped away that your brain doesn't know what to say next. The few simple questions that are left can seem like a very poor meal compared to the rich and varied choices available from the menu above. Rather like the first week of a no-nonsense diet, the mind keeps coming back to the refrigerator door, opening it and gazing longingly at the array of forbidden possibilities inside. There can be a sense of emptiness that seems unnatural and unnecessary as the verbal, left-brain part of the mind struggles to realise that normal patterns of conversation no longer apply.

But there is an obvious purpose to this linguistic minimalism. Let me invite you to try another experiment. Bring to mind an issue you feel rather vulnerable about. Or if you don't have such an issue, just notice what happens inside you when you *think* about having one. Now imagine discussing that issue with three different people; the first might be your mother, the second a respected senior colleague and the third a much-loved but rather difficult friend. Would they all be listening to you in the same way? Would they all be asking you exactly the same questions about your experience? What kind of ideas, assumptions and judgements would each of them bring to the way they listen to you and the questions they ask?

We all live in a world we have spent our whole life creating for ourselves, fully equipped with preconceptions, prejudices, unquestioned assumptions and entrenched beliefs about how that world works. It is impossible for anyone to engage with you without seeing you and hearing you through these filters. As the jazz musician Miles Davis is supposed to have once said, 'If you understood everything I said, you'd be me.' One of the paradoxes of everyday life is that we have to ignore this obvious truth as soon as we start communicating with other people, otherwise we would never get anything done. Then at some point in the day we find something is just not working as we try to communicate with one of these other beings. We may begin to wonder if they are just stupid, or preoccupied, or living in a world of their own. If we are lucky enough to have learned Clean Language, then we not only know that they are indeed living in a world of their own, we can also start making sense of that world, in a way that will probably be as surprising to them as it is to us.

Why? For one thing, Clean Language is made up almost entirely of questions – this means that when you use it, you're finding out things about the other person, not telling them what you think. But even when we ask questions, the questions we ask are usually heavily influenced by the way we see the world and the results we want to get. This is true to a far greater extent than the everyday mind wants to admit. Even when we think we are interpreting a person's words in the most innocent and neutral way, we are almost certainly bringing our own presuppositions to them. Clean questions give you a kind of filter to keep your presuppositions out of the client's space. They do this by focusing entirely on the client's own words (and non-verbal communications), by staying within the logic of the client's world rather than introducing any kind of alternative or competing logic from the therapist's, and by importing no presuppositions into the client's world beyond the simplest concepts like space, time, form and intention.

For example, a woman in a class I was teaching volunteered to do a demonstration with me in which all she had to do was stand in a qi gong posture and notice what happened when she thought about something that was troubling her. After a minute or so, she said she had 'a headachy feeling'. So I asked a Clean question:

What kind of *headachy feeling?*
– A feeling of pressure.

And where in your head is that pressure – in the front, the back, the side, the top?

From the blank look on her face, I could see that I had asked the wrong question, but I couldn't think why. In fact, even she had to stay with the feeling for some time before it started making any sense to her. Then, to her surprise and mine, she said the pressure wasn't coming from inside her head; it was coming from outside, from in front of her.

And that pressure from in front of you is like what?
– A kind of hot wind.

After two more questions, she had translated that vague headachy feeling into a clear understanding that someone important in her life was putting her under much more pressure than she realised.

I had made one slip by asking a question that included my commonsense assumption that a headache must come from somewhere inside her head. But in this case I was wrong. It didn't matter that much, because I was able to ask more Clean questions, ones that helped her to explore her own sense of it in her own way and at her own pace. It's these aspects of experience – the impressions, intuitions, gut feelings, internal shifts and peripheral glimpses that happen in the moment and may not yet have a label or a name – which the verbal mind needs time to comprehend. That is when the mind goes blank – in this woman's case, finding words for the sense of pressure in front of her head. When we use Clean Language in bodywork therapy, it's often all about this space between language and what lies just beyond it, connecting thoughts and feelings so that rather than being separate neurological events, they can fuse together to create new insight.

～ 4 ～

THREE CLEAN QUESTIONS

What is it about Clean Language that helps you and your client get to the heart of an issue so quickly and directly? In Part 2, we look at some scientific research about how mind, brain and body communicate with each other. But for the moment, I'd like to invite you to try it for yourself and just see what happens when you use Clean Language to investigate a physical sensation in your own body. First, let's see what happened for six different people who all tried this exercise themselves, and the surprisingly diverse and vivid responses they got.

To keep it simple, we'll start with the three most basic and versatile Clean Language questions. You can usually help clients make a significant shift in whatever problem they bring to you well before you start any kind of bodywork, using just these three utterly simple questions:

And what kind of…?
And where is…?
And is there anything else about…?

Perhaps you're wondering what's so special about questions like these. You probably ask them all the time in conversations with your clients. But it's what comes after the questions that matters most in Clean Language, and that is what goes on those dotted lines. The keywords and phrases that your client uses are the essential raw material of the whole Clean process. And all you put on that dotted line is your client's exact words, exactly as you heard them. No summarising, no paraphrasing, no changing them to words you're more comfortable with or ones that make more sense to you. Apart from changing the client's 'I' to 'you' and little things that would otherwise sound weird and therefore distracting for the client, you simply keep their words exactly as they are.

So the first step is to choose, from what your client has just said, the keyword or phrase that seems most important. As they talk, it can help to repeat your client's words silently to yourself as if you were recording them. Then listen to the replay in your mind, roll it around in your mouth, embody it, take a moment to get a real sense of how it sounds and how they say it. There's no need to spend much time thinking about what it means. Your brain will do that anyway, but when you start to ask Clean questions, you realise that assuming that you know what the other person means is just a convenient illusion. All you need to do for now is to take that keyword or phrase and put it into one of those very simple questions: '**And what kind of…?**', '**And where is…?**' and '**And is there anything else about…?**'

Notice they all begin with 'And'. You don't always have to begin your Clean question with 'And…', but it's there because it's the Cleanest conjunction you can use. Clean questions are designed to move the client's attention away from normal conversation, even away from the fact that they are talking to you, and instead to focus that attention on their own subjective inner experience. If you say 'And…' you're simply linking your next question with what they've just said, and inviting them to take a further step into that experience. If you say 'But…' or 'So…' you're already introducing a hint of interpretation, or the possibility of another point of view.

Although in many kinds of therapeutic dialogue that other point of view is an essential part of the process, in Clean Language we are doing something radically different. You can always come back to the kind of dialogue you're used to later in the conversation. The point for now is to use Clean questions as 'cleanly' as possible, so you can experience the difference they make. So let's begin.

TRANSFORMING A SYMPTOM

One of the simplest and most common kinds of response, not just with Clean Language but in all forms of mind/body dialogue that focus attention on a symptom, is a change in how the symptom feels. When Lisa asked herself the three Clean questions about one of her own symptoms, she found first that the feeling moved to somewhere else in her body, and then it started to release. Starting with an ache in her left shoulder, she asked:

What kind of *ache in my left shoulder?*
- A hot, burning ache.

And where is *the hot burning ache?*
- Around and under the shoulder blade; it feels trapped.

And *it feels trapped.* **And is there anything else about** *that hot burning ache around and under the shoulder blade?*
- Now it's pinpointing in my side, between the ribs, rather than the shoulder.

Is there anything else about *it pinpointing in your side, between the ribs?*

The response to that question didn't come in words. According to Lisa:

Acknowledging the centre of the pain created a warmth and then a release. The hot burning ache around the scapula lessened considerably and the sharp pain in my side was gone. In myself I felt calmer than I had in days.

She added, 'I found it really interesting how powerful the changes were that I felt by using simple questions to keep my attention on the symptom.'

Thanks to this focused attention, in Lisa's case the response to the questions came first as a sense of heat, then a movement to another part of the body, then a release from the physical sensations and finally that sense of calm.

A METAPHOR FOR CHRONIC PAIN

For Angelika, who lives with the chronic pain of severe arthritis, exploring this pain brought up a metaphor and some strong emotions. Typing her answers into her laptop in a hotel lobby as she asked herself the questions, she wrote:

I sit here in a quiet corner and start the task. I welcome my body, breathing gently, and begin to scan through it, starting with my feet, legs and hips…no complaints (good), and no bad feelings in the back either. Then coming to the chest and shoulders, my breathing stops. I'm aware of really bad pain in my shoulders.

What kind of *really bad pain in my shoulders?*
- It is a heavy pain, like pressure. I start to gulp.

Where exactly is *this heavy pain, like pressure?*
- It seems to be outside me but connected with chains.

And is there anything else about *this heavy pain, like pressure, that's outside me but connected with chains?*
- It feels like a cage. I sit here and I cry silently, my tears are falling on my laptop… I thought it must be easy to be aware of my body; my body is my daily agenda. Surprise; what I actually learned is that the pain is my daily agenda. I sigh, and I'm glad I'm wearing glasses so nobody can see my tears. But soon I start to feel better. I breathe deeply and relax and get the feeling that there is now space between the cage and me. My shoulders and

my neck feel more as if they belong to me rather than to the pain. I will take this feeling into my sleep.

For Angelika, the physical sensations of pain translated themselves into a powerful metaphor, first chains, and then a cage. And notice that, unlike Lisa, she doesn't say that the pain diminished, but that she now feels more space between herself and the cage, and perhaps even more important, a sense of owning this part of her body again, rather than it being owned by the pain.

SLOWING DOWN

In Anna's case, it took only a few Clean questions for her to be able to turn an unexplained feeling of nausea into clear advice in simple words that popped into her head. After a very busy day, she started asking herself the Clean questions just after her evening meal:

- I felt into my body and became aware of a feeling of nausea and tightness.

And where is that feeling of nausea and tightness?
- Around the solar plexus area.

And is there anything else about that feeling of nausea and tightness around the solar plexus area?
- A strong feeling of there not being enough room to move, both within my body and around my body.

And is there anything else about there not being enough room to move?
- These words come to me: 'I need to make more time and space in my life for food.'

She continued to take deep breaths until the restriction eased. Then she realised that although she didn't have to eat her dinner in a hurry that evening: 'I'd carried the time pressure I had been under in the day into the mealtime. The experience made me consider how, when my life is busy, everything speeds up.'

So for Anna, the questions turned an undefined nausea into a clear message to herself about slowing down. Once she was able to eat at the pace that was right for her body, her body responded by releasing that feeling of there not being enough room to move.

A POISONED FEELING

For Gerry, the Clean questions brought a real learning about how much information there can be in a symptom he not only thought he understood perfectly, but actually felt rather ashamed of:

Yesterday I was recovering from some serious drinking at a party the night before. I asked myself, '**What kind of** *hangover is this?*'
- It's a poisoned feeling; my body is sluggish and tired, with a dry throat.

Where exactly is *that poisoned feeling?*
- At the back of the mouth, which feels very dry.

Is there anything else about *that poisoned feeling at the back of the mouth, which feels very dry?*
- I have an ache in my upper back – a long-term thing that is often affected by emotional stress.

The party I had been to was an annual family get-together but lots of grief had been stirred up because of the recent death of a family member. I think I was holding it in my back. In fact, the feeling taps into quite early childhood feelings of vulnerability. As I asked myself the questions, it allowed me to engage with the feelings and isolate them in their component parts. I felt more engaged with my body rather than just passively accepting a feeling of being ill. I was amazed at how much information came up from what I had initially dismissed as a mild sickness induced by overindulgence.

Gerry's story is a good example of how the questions can take you very deeply very quickly into surprisingly emotional territory.

WHEN TO BACK OFF

For Nishat, this was also true, and she learned something valuable from it:

- It took me a while to settle into a space in my mind to be able to ask and answer the Clean questions, as I realised how out of touch with my body I have been. Once I started the questions it really surprised me how quickly they cut to the core and I got a clear picture of what I needed for my body – it was quite outstanding. Let's say that the questions really helped me focus and be true to myself, in a gentle way. I felt a tightness and stiffness in the whole of my back but particularly inside and behind my left scapula, like my heart was sore.

And what kind of tightness and stiffness was this?
- Like armouring, solid and protective.

Anything else about this tightness and stiffness, like armouring?
- I found that the tightness and stiffness made it difficult for me to take a deep breath in and realised when I tried to that it connected to something I was not ready to deal with. The whole exercise made me stand up and twist and stretch and massage my spine, and at the end take much-needed deep and satisfying breaths right down into my abdomen.

Nishat did something very sensible here, which anyone who starts asking Clean questions should remember. Because they can go so deep so fast, it's very important to acknowledge when you or your client get to a place that doesn't feel ready to be dealt with. Respect the information, in whatever form it comes, and back off gently. As Nishat did, it can be very helpful at that point to shift from verbal questioning to movement or bodywork.

THE POWER OF METAPHOR

Finally, Janet was also taken by surprise at how quickly a metaphor emerged from her physical symptom, and at the strength of her emotional reaction. The part of her body that drew her attention was 'Something in my upper chest'.

And what kind of something is that something in your upper chest?
- It feels like a piece of wood, a door.

And is there anything else about that door?
- A closed, shut door without any glass.

And is there anything else about a closed shut door without any glass in your upper chest?
- It aches and feels heavy, pulling my neck and shoulder down.

And is there anything else about pulling my neck and shoulder down?
- It becomes dark and scary like a cave; my heart is pounding.

And is there anything else about dark and scary?

The next bit took a while to come…

- It's something I'm carrying.

Rather than go into a new line of questioning about this 'something' she was carrying, Janet chose to go back to the original symptom to see how it had changed.

And when it's something I'm carrying, how is that something in my upper chest now?
- Less achy and closed – I need to move and stretch it.

She commented, 'It was very interesting how quickly I got from a visual description – "closed door" – to "dark and scary". Then it sort of stuck and I couldn't seem to get any further. The next morning, though, my chest felt fine.'

So even though she found the questions taking her to somewhere quite frightening, and her heart was actually pounding, she felt safe enough to stay with the process and acknowledge that 'It's something I'm carrying'. Of course, the fact that her chest felt fine the next morning doesn't mean that the problem is resolved or won't come back. It might have felt fine anyway, whether she asked Clean questions or not. But it's worth noticing from her experience that you don't have to go on asking Clean questions until you get an 'explanation' of what's behind the symptom. Like Nishat, she found the right place to let the body's way of processing take over, using movement and stretching. As the practitioner, when you think your client may have got to this point, you can check by asking '**And is there anything else...?**' and if the answer comes as a desire to move, stretch, stand up or lie down, then ask them if they want to explore that in their own way, or if that's a good place to start working directly with whatever kind of bodywork you do. Whichever they choose, you can continue to ask more Clean questions if that seems appropriate.

So there's your first example of Clean Language in action – how a few simple questions can quickly take you well beyond the familiar labels you might have for a symptom, reversing the way the verbal mind expects to work. Instead of using words as tools to project ideas out into the world and, via other people's brains, to make things happen, Clean questions take your words and follow them back into your brain and body, your nervous system and connective tissues, muscles, organs, nerves and bones, and into the 'psycho-geography' of the spaces inside you and around you. Somehow from there, new words or images emerge, to pop into an often-bewildered brain. Just as silences in conversation can feel awkward, the verbal mind is not happy when there are no words to describe what's going on. To learn how to ask Clean questions effectively, you need to allow that sense of bewilderment to become familiar and comfortable. So the challenge in the next two chapters is to do what these practitioners did, and try these three Clean questions on yourself.

~ 5 ~

CLEAN QUESTIONS FOR
A COLD SHOULDER

So if you're ready, I'd like to invite you to try it for yourself and just see what happens when you use Clean Language to investigate a physical sensation in your own body. Clean Language is very easy to learn compared to most languages, but when we use it as a way of communicating with the body, the real challenge is in learning that the body thinks and communicates in very different ways from the ones the normal, everyday verbal mind is used to. That's why it's so important to try it for yourself. When you do, you begin to realise that asking yourself Clean questions can become a very useful reflective practice, a kind of mind/body meditation. But if you're still not sure about how to do it, I'll give you an example of how I might use the questions with a symptom of my own, just as I would with a client, exploring it as sensitively and in as much depth as I can as a preparation for moving into the bodywork part of the session.

I'll use those first three questions you already know:

And what kind of...?
And where is...?
And is there anything else about...?

As you follow the transcript, you might want to read the questions out loud to yourself, just to let them sink in. And one more thing – when you're using Clean Language for mind/body therapy, it's best if both you and your client take some time to loosen up, settle down and have a meditative moment to reconnect to your sense of your body and breath. So take a minute to get comfortable, because the more comfortable you are as you read this, the more comfortable I will be about exploring my own private interior world with a complete stranger. Okay? Thank you.

My symptom is a stuck feeling in my right shoulder, which I've had for the past three days, since I cycled home after work on the first cold night of autumn, still wearing summer clothes and without a scarf or gloves. What's bothering me about it is that even though I've been doing all the right things to get rid of it – applying gentle heat, doing qi gong, stretching, drinking ginger tea and so on – it's stubbornly resisting my efforts to make it go away. This is exactly the sort of situation in which a bit of Clean Language can help.

So, the keywords I will pick from all that are 'A stuck feeling in my right shoulder.' I'll also pick the bit about 'stubbornly resisting', since that sounds like an important hint about the relationship between the symptom and its owner. And since the owner is me, and stubborn resistance can be irritating, and I am indeed a bit irritated with it now, I'd better take a step back, stop trying to get rid of it and engage my curiosity instead, with the help of a few Clean questions.

*And when there's a stuck feeling in my right shoulder that's stubbornly resisting me, **what kind of** stuck feeling **is that**?*

Funny – as soon as I ask that, I start noticing how cold my right shoulder feels, cold as well as stuck. To answer the question, I have to move it around a little and bend my neck over to the left to really feel the stuckness.

- It's a kind of hunched, defensive stuckness, and I notice how cold it feels.

Hmmm… I can't stop my brain from noticing that while 'cold' is a simple elemental kind of thing, 'hunched' and 'defensive' sound more like reactions to some kind of threat. But the point is not to analyse or think it through. You can't stop these thoughts popping into your head as you hear your client's answers, but it's best to clear them from your mind before you ask the next Clean question, '**And where is…?**' This question is so important in any kind of mind/body therapy because the body speaks such a different language from the verbal mind. Though the mind can be anywhere instantly, the body has to be in one place at a time, so knowing where it is, and where it is in relation to other things, is tremendously important to it. Asking the '**Where…?**' question really helps the mind to understand this.

Since I already know where the symptom is, I'll ask a slightly different version:

And where exactly is that hunched, defensive stuckness that feels cold?

Notice I've included in this second question all the keywords that have come in answer to the first one, because I don't know which one of those keywords will get the strongest response from the original symptom. What I am aiming for is a question that makes something go 'ping' not just in my mind but also in some way that is felt physically, no matter how subtle that feeling may be. To answer the question, I have to focus my attention more precisely on where the ache is, and that in itself already creates a sense of something about to change.

In this case, the word 'cold' seems to be what does it. When I hear it repeated back, I feel a kind of constriction or tightening in my shoulder. It goes all the way through the muscle at the top of the shoulder blade. As a professional bodyworker, you might be tempted to say 'Trapezius' but when you're asking or answering Clean questions it's best to avoid technical language. Bodies don't speak Latin, and I've only ever had one client who could.

So I'm ready to ask my next Clean question, the '**Anything else…?**' one:

And is there anything else about this hunched, defensive, cold feeling that goes all the way through the muscle on the top of the shoulder blade?

Again, I'm using several keywords, and you may think it sounds a bit repetitive or pedantic, but the point is not what it sounds like to the verbal, logical mind; the mind I'm trying to reach is the bodymind, the one that knows a lot more than the verbal mind about why this symptom hasn't gone away yet.

– It's a kind of freezing stiffness.

I'm surprised by the word 'freezing' – that sounds a bit extreme, but it's important not to interrogate or censor the response that comes out – just let the Clean questions do their work. So I've asked all three questions; now I can choose any one of them to continue my investigations:

A *freezing stiffness.* **And where exactly is** *that freezing stiffness?*
– All round the back of my shoulder.

As I focus on it I start to feel my right shoulder moving forwards and this soon turns into a movement of my whole arm. Like a kind of gentle self-hypnosis, I feel my elbow wanting to move, my fingers opening and the whole configuration of my upper arm and shoulder muscles changing. Holding my arm in that position, I let my left arm mirror it, because it seems to want to. Now I'm in a kind of qi gong posture, as if my arms are wrapped around a big ball in front of my chest, and finally I get some evidence that the Clean questions are working – my shoulder is starting to feel warmer. When I test it by bending my neck to the left again, there's less tightness and more flexibility in the knot of muscle there. This is good. It's as if my bodymind, as soon as it thinks that I'm really listening to it, is only too happy to show me exactly what it wants me to do. Instead of imposing a standard sequence of movements and stretches on it as I did in my previous attempts to get rid of the symptom, it's now guiding me to listen to what this 'stubborn' symptom is trying to tell me. I do this all the time with my clients, so why does it take me so long to remember to do it with myself? As a practitioner yourself, I'm sure you've been here too, so let's get on with the questions:

And when it feels warmer in your right shoulder, and there's more flexibility, is there anything else about warmer and more flexibility?

I hold my arms in that position, and take a deeper breath – almost a sigh. As I breathe in, an image of my ribs flashes through my mind, seen from the inside, as if they're covered in frost, and I realise that the tightening has an emotional quality, a hint of fear. Maybe it's a tightening against the oncoming cold of winter. Being skinny, I'm vulnerable to cold weather, and last winter was the coldest in England since records began. It was also a time when I was feeling vulnerable in other ways. My father's death earlier in the year had left me feeling depressed and anxious, and I remember how the cold sometimes got to my bones in a way that made me acutely aware of my own mortality. No wonder there was a 'hunched, defensive' quality to the stiffness in my shoulder. As this whole train of thought passes through my mind, the tension in my ribs relaxes and the glowing image of a crackling fire appears in my mind's eye.

Could this cosy image be my bodymind telling me that I'm finally beginning to get the message? Time for one more Clean question:

And is there anything else about a crackling fire?

Immediately I notice myself take a deeper breath and see a warm internal flame inside my ribs, more or less where my heart should be. I sit for a while silently, not trying to make things happen, but very aware of the image of the flame. My attention drifts away for a while into dream-like thoughts, then returns to this flame, as if by giving it my attention, I'm giving it more oxygen. Perhaps this is part of the message behind my stubborn symptom – that there's some emotional thawing-out still to do, in relation to my father's death. My arms, still held out in front of me, want to move up higher, opposite my chest, and to stretch out gently, opening the space between my shoulder blades in my upper back, which in turn gives me a sense of relaxing around the heart.

So, as often happens with Clean Language, just a few questions, and a bit of willingness to listen to my body, have helped me get to a much deeper understanding of my apparently straightforward physical symptom. Not only does its refusal to respond to my efforts to make it go away now make perfect sense, it has also given me some guidance on what I need to do to release that stubborn stiffness and restore my shoulder to free and easy movement. Not bad for just six questions!

You may be wondering, if a client came to see you for a bodywork session and you'd helped them get this far with Clean questions, what would you do next? How exactly do you make the transition into whatever kind of bodywork you do? And how much time can you spend asking Clean questions before you have to start doing your usual kind of treatment? In Part 3, we'll look at that kind of question in more detail, but for the moment there are two things to remember. The first is that you *have already been* working with the body. With Clean questions, you have brought the bodymind into the conversation, and it has been communicating in its own way. By using Clean Language, you have already connected with aspects of your client's being that can only be reached through the bodymind – the animal intelligence that knows about space and safety, and the somatic intelligence that expresses itself through movement, metaphor and 'felt sense'. Any intervention you make now will benefit from the trust you have built at that deep level, thanks to Clean questions and your Clean listening.

The second thing to remember is that there doesn't have to be any direct or obvious connection at all between what has come up in your Clean conversation and what seems appropriate in the bodywork part of the session. This will vary from therapy to therapy, but it can be just as effective to forget all about those keywords and phrases while you focus on your treatment in the normal way, leaving it up to the client to make their own connections. Sometimes a little prompting can help: for example, asking some questions at the end of the session to find out how your client is now and simply reminding them (check your notes if you need to) of the keywords they started out with. In the case of me and my shoulder, at the end of the treatment a practitioner might ask:

And how are you now?
- Good. Quite light actually, all through my whole body.

And is there anything else about quite light all through your whole body?
- I feel really grounded at the same time.

And when you're quite light all through your whole body, and you feel really grounded at the same time, how is your right shoulder now?
- (Moving the shoulder to check) Still there a bit, but a lot better. Like there's more space inside the joint.

And is there anything else about more space inside the joint?
- Yeah. When I breathe, my chest feels more relaxed, warmer actually. It's like someone's switched the central heating on.

And is there anything else about switched the central heating on?
- It's like my arms want to lift up again like they did before. That's what switches the heating on.
  (Pausing for a few breaths) And then the stiff feeling's completely gone!

And would allowing your arms to lift up like that be a good thing to practise until our next session?
- Yes.

In this way, at the end of the session your questions can be a helpful way to confirm to the client's everyday mind that something really has changed in relation to the original problem. It's also a good way to help the client's own bodymind suggest some 'homework' – like this spontaneous suggestion from my bodymind of a qi gong posture for my arms that they can do to build on the effects of the treatment.

~ 6 ~

LETTING YOUR BODY
ANSWER BACK

Are you ready to try this – to ask those three simple questions about something you're aware of in your body right now? I strongly suggest that you resist the temptation just to read through this next part without actually trying the questions out. Why? Because strange things happen when you ask Clean questions – even to yourself – and to be able to help your clients with them, it's important to have experienced these very subjective cognitive and somatic shifts, and how feelings, sounds, words, images and metaphors can all be involved. And if you still don't want to try it just now, read this chapter anyway, because you'll find some useful hints along the way.

If you want to listen to your somatic self, it helps to make a few preparations to your position. In a normal Clean Language session, you wouldn't tell your client how to sit, since the way they occupy the chair is an intimate portrayal of their habitual posture, an essential truth about who they are and how they are, and if it changes as you ask Clean questions, that in itself is useful information for you both. But for the purposes of this exercise, it helps to let your body know that you're planning to pay attention to it. So get yourself comfortable and if you're sitting down, it usually helps to have the soles of both feet on the floor. If you're used to meditating, a loose version of your favourite meditation posture might be a good way to start, but if you find your body wanting to move, then allow that to happen. Breathe easily, just noticing the feeling of breath coming in and out, without forcing your breath to be deeper, slower or anything else. Now begin to notice what you're aware of in your body. Maybe it's obvious – some tension somewhere that you're immediately aware of, or maybe an ache that's been there for days, or a tight muscle that's so familiar that it feels like it's a normal part of how you are. Or maybe you're not aware of anything in particular, at least not yet. Take your time…once you begin to pay attention to the body, you have to be prepared to communicate with it in its own language and its own way, and time is one of the things the body does differently from the everyday clock-conscious mind. The body knows time in terms of how long it takes to breathe in and out or how fast or slow your heart is beating, or by the rhythms of morning and evening or the menstrual cycle – it's not so interested in the ticking of the clock, though it knows about that too. If you're not aware of anything obvious, just come back to your breathing and wait. It doesn't help to go searching for symptoms – wait for one to come to you.

When you find something, notice how you're aware of it and what words – if any – you can describe it with. Some feelings are quite difficult to put into words, and by trying to describe them in words that don't really fit, you already change your relationship to the sensation itself. So keep your language vague if the feeling is vague: 'Something in my right thigh', or even, 'I don't really know', is all you need to get started.

Then you're ready for the first Clean question:

And what kind of…?

When you put your keywords into the space with the dots, notice something odd can happen to the way the sentence sounds.

A Clean question aims to use the client's keywords as exactly as possible – and at the moment, the client is you, so just put your own words into the question, for example:

And what kind of something in my right thigh? or
And what kind of I don't really know?

Notice '**What kind of…?**' is a completely open and flexible question, which is what makes it so useful as a way to start. It doesn't invite 'Yes or No' answers, it simply directs your attention more precisely to the feeling itself. This is so important because one of our main aims in using Clean Language in mind/body therapy is to find the words that lead us deeper into felt experience, not away from it. If a client said, 'I've been getting an ache in my wrist' and you then asked, 'Does it feel like arthritis?' notice the effect of that question, compared to simply saying, 'An ache in your wrist? What kind of ache?' The question about arthritis invites a straightforward 'Yes' or 'No' and is about what label to give the feeling and how to categorise it – important from a diagnostic point of view but not what you're trying to do when you ask Clean questions. By contrast, 'What kind of ache?' invites you to focus your attention and curiosity on the feeling itself.

If you've been reading this as well as focusing on what you're aware of in your own body, you'll have probably already noticed some shift or response there as you ask the '**What kind of…?**' question. If not, try it now, and notice what happens to your awareness of it, and what words come in answer to the question.

These are the words you now put into your second Clean question – an absolutely vital one for mind/body work – one which may sound very obvious but can deliver some surprisingly powerful results:

And where is…? or
And where exactly is…?

Again, as you ask yourself this, notice the response, including non-verbal ones like a spontaneous wish to move, stretch or flex a joint, twitches, tingles, gurgles in the belly and so on. The '**Where....?**' question focuses awareness more precisely, often setting up a kind of loop of neurological information flow that can start to set changes in motion.

Now if you're ready for the third of our basic Clean questions, notice again the words that come to describe what you're aware of now, and then thread those words into the following question:

And is there anything else about...?

Notice again how invitingly open this question is, drawing no conclusions, making no suggestions about meaning or interpretation, simply encouraging you to take one step further in this process of communicating with your own body in a kind of language which it understands and can respond to.

Now that you've been through the first cycle of questions, and tried out all three of them, you're free to experiment. Just go on asking the questions, in any order you like; or if in doubt, just go on asking '**And is there anything else about...?**' again and again, bringing your attention back each time to that original symptom to see whether it responds, and if so, how.

I'll wait while you try it...

How did you do? If you're not the kind of person who tries out exercises as you read them, then you could get a friend to ask you the questions. The advantage of asking yourself these questions, though, is that you can go entirely at your own pace, you can give yourself as much commentary as you like on what you're experiencing as you go, and you don't have to pay any attention or devote any of your precious neurological circuitry to all the fine-tuned interactions that arise simply from having to talk to someone else. Of course, one of the main reasons for using Clean Language is to reduce those interactions to a minimum for the client, to create a different kind of space, a 'cleaner' space, in which different kinds of answers can come. But the space you give yourself is very different from the space that can exist between two people, and it's good to experience that before moving on to practising your Clean questions with someone else.

And when you do, you'll probably find – like Angelika with her poignant example of a 'cage' of chronic pain, or Janet, who was surprised at how quickly she found herself in front of 'a closed, shut door without any glass', or me with my 'crackling fire' and a 'warm internal flame' – that your mind and your body share at least one common currency, and that is the language of metaphor. Metaphor is not only a vital part of mind/body communication, it is also the place where Clean Language began, so before you go on to learn more Clean questions, we need to look at why it's so important to listen carefully to the metaphors your clients offer you.

$\sim 7 \sim$

MIND, MATTER AND METAPHOR

A cyclist recovering from a head-on collision with a motorcyclist delivering pizzas says the pain of breaking her leg was, 'like a thousand burning hot splinters running through my body at a million miles an hour'. She could have just said it was agonising or excruciating. What was so important to her about finding such a vivid way to express the felt experience? An elderly client winces when I lightly touch a certain point; brought back from semi-consciousness, he suddenly announces in a booming voice, 'That's an odd, hopeless pain.' Another client, who has been told by her doctor that she has only a few months to live, says, 'I feel like I'm rotting from the inside out.' A young man starting a new relationship says his severe panic attacks are, 'bringing up a shitload of stuff from the past'. When a client says something like this in the middle of a treatment, what do you do? Maybe acknowledge it with an understanding 'Hmm' while trying to stay focused on the bodywork, or maybe even start a mental search for diagnostic clues in what they say? I often find myself doing both, until I remind myself to accept it for what it is – a metaphor – and to get curious about what it may have to offer.

Listening to the way your clients talk about their problems and symptoms, and how they phrase their outcomes, you will notice they use all kinds of metaphors. The most obvious are the ones expressed in words, but they may also be expressed through gesture, movement or posture. Whether verbal or physical, these metaphors will almost certainly be out of the client's awareness as they make them. They will often be out of your own awareness too, since you have plenty of other things to focus on as you gather the information you need to make some kind of diagnosis and plan a treatment. But all these kinds of metaphor can provide a direct pathway into your client's subjective psychosomatic reality – a path that is usually easy to follow if you ask a few Clean questions. But most metaphors are so deeply embedded in everyday language that we barely notice them in use ('deeply embedded', for example, is a metaphor). Learning to recognise them is the first step, so let's begin by looking at the three essential characteristics which make up any kind of metaphor.

DESCRIBING ONE THING IN TERMS OF ANOTHER

Metaphors have an unusual power to communicate and motivate and one reason for that is that they are almost always built around one clear, strong image. If a football commentator talks about putting the ball 'in the back of the net', there's a satisfying sense of knowing exactly what that means – the expression has a more visual and visceral 'kick' to it than if they had just talked about 'scoring a goal'. Of course, it's not a metaphor yet – it's literally true that the ball went into the back of the net. But if a doctor uses the same expression to motivate a soccer-loving patient to finish a course of medication – 'When you start taking it you're tackling the illness; but you have to finish the whole pack to get the ball into the back of the net' – then it's a metaphor. Why? Because it transfers that original strong image from one context to another.

If you go to Athens you will see vans go by with 'metaphoriki' written on them (in Greek letters, of course). These vans are not full of metaphors – 'metaphoriki' is Greek for 'removals' and this is what metaphors do. They remove one experience and carry it across to another context; the Greek origin of the word comes from 'meta' (meaning *across* or *over*) and 'phor' (meaning *to carry*). Meaning is 'carried across' by describing one thing – literally – in terms of another.

DESCRIBING THE ABSTRACT IN TERMS OF THE FAMILIAR

The second key characteristic of metaphors is that they tend to describe something abstract or complex in terms of something familiar and simple. Good science writers know how to translate extremely complex notions into images that seem to make sense – 'black holes', 'the big bang' and 'dark matter' are all easy-to-grasp images for phenomena which are by definition beyond the bounds of all human experience. In this way, metaphors usually describe something abstract in terms of something you can experience directly through your senses. Our everyday language is full of micro-metaphors of exactly this kind, difficult to spot because they're in such constant use. For example, if you say a person is 'hard' to get to know, you're describing your experience of them in terms of a basic tactile sense of something that doesn't give way easily. The subtle psychological detail of your encounter with that person is depicted as an easy-to-understand felt sense. To call someone 'soft in the head' is not the same as calling them 'soft-hearted', yet neither makes any sense at all unless you have some idea of what softness *feels* like.

In mind/body work, metaphors can translate complex psycho-physiological processes into something easier to grasp. Clients may use very familiar expressions like, 'I'm still digesting the news', or 'My heart missed a beat', or offer their own freshly coined phrases.

For example, the following three sentences are all things clients have said to me to describe things they experienced during a treatment:

'My head filled up with light.'

'It feels like I have tiny fish swimming in my legs.'

'I was in a bubble where there was no time or space.'

Even though these are all describing subjective and unfamiliar experiences, they are doing it with the image of something familiar – 'light', 'fish', 'bubble'.

METAPHORS CONDENSE INFORMATION

The third key characteristic of metaphors is that they can *condense* an immense range of information into a few words or a single image. When you meet a metaphor, it's easy to forget just how condensed it is, especially if it sounds like a familiar one. The temptation can be to assume that the meaning is obvious and to want to move on beyond this well-worn figure of speech, but the art of Clean Language lies in recognising that the metaphor itself, however clichéd it may sound, is (to use another cliché) an offer you can't refuse. As soon as you pay it the courtesy of stopping to say hello and asking a few simple questions, it will often reveal to you layers of meaning that neither you nor the client had any idea of. We have seen plenty of examples already of how rich they can be. So making a point of inquiring about these metaphors is a good way of training your clients to be more curious about what their own bodymind may be trying to tell them, and opening up a pathway of communication between their inner world and their everyday conscious mind.

Such training is best done step by step, at the client's own pace. The results may not be dramatic, but you are building an evidence base for them, session by session, that the metaphors they think with can have deep somatic roots. For example, a client once showed me the importance – when it comes to metaphor – of accepting whatever is offered. For several sessions he had been intensely focused on issues from the past, in a way that seemed to me that he was almost trapped in his own story, even finding it difficult to answer my questions about what he might want from the treatment since that involved thinking about the future. After a few sessions, this started to loosen up and he began this particular one by saying that things were beginning to change. When I asked what kind of change, he said, 'New horizons beckon'. For a moment, I was actually slightly disappointed that after several sessions of patient work, this well-worn phrase was the best he could come up with. I was tempted to ignore the cliché and ask again what kind of changes he was noticing in his life. But I paused and reminded myself that I actually had no idea what these new horizons were really like for him. So I asked, 'And what kind of new horizons beckon?', expecting him to zoom in on some tantalising future possibility (a good example of how you can be Clean with your question but not so Clean with what you're hoping that question will achieve). The client looked a bit baffled, but after a few moments' contemplation what he said surprised me: 'The new horizons still seem far away'. I felt my bubble of momentum punctured, recognised it as mine, not his, and realised that what was important for *him* about these new horizons was not what was on them, but how distant they seemed. When I asked, '**And is there anything else about** new horizons that still seem far away?' he stared for quite a long time into the distance, hardly breathing, then sighed, and something softened around the centre of his chest as he said, 'It's just nice to know they're there'. For me, that somatic softening was proof that his metaphor was not just linguistic decoration, and when I drew his attention to it by asking '**And what just happened?**' he became aware of that softening too.

According to Wendy Sullivan and Judy Rees in their book *Clean Language: Revealing Metaphors and Opening Minds* (2008, p.19), metaphor is 'at the heart of the Clean way of thinking'. Metaphors show us how we make sense of the world and they provide the map by which we navigate our way through it. As bodywork practitioners, our clients' metaphors are a particular gift; not just linguistic frills, but more like the end of a thread which, followed carefully, with the simplest and most open kind of questions, can lead us to the patterns that underlie both their symptoms and ways we might discover to resolve them.

~ 8 ~

EMBODIED LANGUAGE,
EMBODIED MIND

The sculptor Antony Gormley has achieved worldwide success with his life-size statues of his own body. To make them, he has to stay completely still, eyes closed, putting his absolute trust in his artist wife, Vicken Parsons, as she wraps him first in a protective layer of clingfilm and then covers him in gluey patches of material which gradually dry hard around him, leaving him – apart from a tube to breathe through – completely encased and immobilised. The inspiration to use his own body as his subject matter came from his long-term practice of meditation. 'The casting process takes about an hour and a half,' he explains, 'and I think this is the main way in which my training in meditation has fed into my work. It depends on total concentration on maintaining stillness' (Gormley 2011). His sculptures certainly reflect that stillness and that meditative quality. 'The body is the root of all our experience,' he says; 'through it all our impressions of the world come and from it all we have to share with the world is expressed.'[1]

---

1   Antony Gormley, from the plaque on his sculpture 'Transport', Canterbury Cathedral, Canterbury.

This may sound obvious (if we remember that the head is part of the body), but it's only comparatively recently that academic philosophers and psychologists have begun to take the idea seriously. In her book *Consciousness in Action* (1998), the philosopher Susan Hurley was one of the first to look beyond what she called the conventional 'sandwich' model of cognition, in which one slice of bread corresponds to our perceptual input, the other slice to our behavioural output, while between them, the filling of the sandwich, is the brain. In this model, all our thinking about what we perceive and about how to respond to what we perceive happens inside the head. The sense of the mind as being somehow independent of the body is so powerful in Western culture that it is hard even to find language to describe how mind and body might be seen as part of one system.

But the relatively new academic field of embodied cognition rejects this notion of the mind as a sort of skull-bound computer. Instead it suggests that the fact that we live in human bodies determines everything about the way we perceive and understand the world. As the two original pioneers of embodied cognition, George Lakoff and Mark Johnson, point out in their book *Philosophy in the Flesh* (1999, p.266), 'There is no mind separate from and independent of the body, nor are there thoughts that have an existence independent of bodies and brains.' They take the etymological micro-metaphors of which language is made up as evidence for this; for example, even a field as apparently abstract as mathematics has its roots in the ten digits of the human hand.

How does this relate to metaphor? In many of the metaphors we take for granted, we find physical experience being used to describe more complex emotional and relational things. The idea of affection, for example, is conveyed by the bodily sensation of warmth, as in 'a warm welcome' or 'a warm smile', while an unfriendly person is 'cold'. In another metaphorical temperature zone, though, someone who can keep their head in a stressful situation is 'cool', while someone who acts on impulse is 'hot-headed'. Especially in mind/body work, it is vital to note that metaphors don't just come in words – the way a client uses space and movement can be metaphorical too; happiness is conveyed in gesture, posture and language as 'up', sadness as 'down'. And when we finally understand a difficult concept we say we've 'got it', as if we can hold it in our hands. From these clues, we see how our early sensorimotor and emotional experience of movement, space and relationship gives rise to the primary metaphorical frameworks with which we think.

Another source of clues is in the structure of the brain itself. This metaphorical 'carrying across' can be seen in the way that parts of the brain which register bodily sensation influence parts which are responsible for emotional response. As neuroscientist David J. Linden says in his book *Touch: The Science of Hand, Heart and Mind* (2015, p.174), 'Everyday language is reflective of neural processes. The similarity of emotional pain and physical pain is not merely a construction of evocative or poetic speech. The metaphor is real and it is embedded in the brain's emotional pain circuitry.' As the poet William Blake put it, with more neurological accuracy than he could have known, 'Each outcry of the hunted Hare/A fiber from the Brain does tear' (Erdman 2008, p.493). And psychiatrist Dan Siegel in his book *Mindsight* (2010, p.195) notes, 'The pain of social rejection is mediated in an area of the middle pre-frontal cortex that also registers physical pain from a bodily injury. That area is called the Anterior Cingulate Cortex and it straddles the boundary between thinking cortex and feeling limbic. It also… plays a key role in the resonance circuitry that lets us feel connected to others and to ourselves.' So social rejection really *is* painful, as far as our bodymind is concerned.

Embodied cognition takes metaphor very seriously, seeing language essentially as something that has evolved by taking the known and familiar and using it to describe the abstract and conceptual. As bodywork therapists we know from experience how much information the body stores outside the brain, and how much a simple change in movement or posture can change the way we think. When we use Clean questions in bodywork therapy, we're inviting the everyday verbal mind, which operates mainly through abstract categories and concepts, to find language for the bodymind's moment-to-moment flow of felt experience. No wonder that the verbal mind's first response is often silence, as it searches for words that may be hard to find.

In bodywork, we may start with things the client considers are purely physical problems but when we work carefully and patiently with Clean questions, there usually comes a point when all the body's hints and symptoms suddenly transform into something that the thinking mind can recognise as a kind of 'carrying across' from the tangibly physical into the emotional, relational and cognitive realms. Maybe the swirl of a hand turns into a sense of 'flow', or a straightening of the spine becomes 'Actually, I think I can do this'. But even when metaphors appear in the form of archetypes or animal imagery, the Brothers Grimm or *The Sound of Music*, this does not mean that as bodywork practitioners we are (to use a metaphor) 'out of our depth'. In fact, Clean Language provides us with exactly the tools we need to help clients make their own sense of these things, and to incorporate them usefully into their experience of bodywork and their everyday life.

∽ 9 ∽

HOW DOES IT WORK AND
WHERE DOES IT COME FROM?

You could sum up in two simple steps what we do when we use Clean Language. First, you use as exactly as possible the words that are offered to you by your client, and second, you offer these words back to your client in a set of simple, open questions. Sooner or later, if your client is willing to play the Clean game with you at all, they will offer you a metaphor, maybe an obvious one like, 'My shoulder is on fire', or maybe one more hidden like, 'I just want to be clear about my options'. We saw in the last two chapters how metaphor is like the connective tissue of language, the thing that holds it all together, and that most of the metaphors we use are woven so deeply into the fabric of everyday language that we can easily pass them by. I managed at least three metaphors in that last sentence – how many did you notice? One reason why Clean Language works is because it gives us a way to take a client's metaphors seriously – literally in fact – and to begin a respectful, patient, even playful exploration of where they go. To understand why Clean Language takes metaphor so seriously, let's look at the work of the man who developed it, David Grove.

DAVID GROVE

People who have suffered some kind of trauma often find that what they experienced becomes literally unspeakable, even to a therapist. Trauma expert Peter Levine, in his book *Waking the Tiger* (1997), sees in the Greek myth of Medusa a powerful analogy for this phenomenon. If you looked into her eyes you would be turned to stone, just as a trauma victim may again feel paralysed and frozen when asked to go back into that traumatic event. To defeat Medusa, Perseus had to look at her only through her reflection in his polished shield. In Somatic Experiencing therapy, Levine creates a safe space in which the client is able to release the trauma via the way it has come to be reflected in their own body. In the same way, New Zealand-born psychotherapist David Grove, working with traumatised clients in the 1980s, noticed that while they found it difficult or impossible to speak about their traumatic experience directly, they often used metaphor as a way of reflecting that experience so that it could be safely expressed and worked with. A woman who suffered abuse as a child, for example, might find a chronic abdominal pain turning into 'a poisonous cloud that can't get out'.

Like other therapists working with the therapeutic power of metaphor at the time, he discovered that they often had a logic of their own that held the key to resolving the unresolved energies, emotions and cognitions of that traumatic experience. The second thing he discovered was that his own well-intentioned attempts as a therapist to understand and interpret these metaphors were somehow getting in the way of or distorting his client's internal process. How could he help the client explore this inner metaphorical landscape without importing his own constructs and intentions? It was this challenge that led him to start searching for the kind of questions that would eventually become Clean Language.

As a psychotherapist, he was clearly fascinated by the language of metaphor, but at the same time he seems to have been acutely sensitive to the possibility that these kinds of metaphors might have somatic roots – that metaphor might be one of the key ways that the cognitive mind and the bodymind communicate. There seemed to be a direct link between the words and images the client used and the way the trauma was somatically stored inside them. As Peter Levine puts it, as a client begins to release a traumatic memory, 'Something that feels internally like a rock, for example, may suddenly seem to melt into a warm liquid' (Levine 1997, p.253).

MAKING TRAUMA SAFE TO EXPLORE

As bodywork therapists, we have some advantages in working with trauma, because so much of its effect is embedded in the body's tissues and energetic field. Trauma by definition overwhelms the conscious mind's ability to process the traumatic experience, so while trying to resolve it cognitively – for example, by training the client to deliberately practise new mental habits – may help them to manage their symptoms better, it is unlikely to change its somatic imprint. But trying to resolve trauma purely through bodywork can also have its limits if the mind is not involved. Grove was looking for a way to help clients safely explore this mind/body link that metaphors seemed to offer, and it's interesting to see just how viscerally aware his language is, for example in this passage about how he came up with this new way of asking questions:

> Clean questions only ask questions which feel right, are easily answered and have the physical sense that the answer is coming from within the metaphor itself. If the metaphor is a rock in the stomach, a clean question feels as if it is going to the stomach and being answered by the stomach, rather than going through the ears and being processed by the brain. (Grove 2010)

So what is it about Clean Language that makes it such a useful tool for cultivating this kind of mind/body awareness? It is not just the questions themselves – most of them are perfectly normal ones that you might well hear in any conversation. Nor is the emphasis on leaving space for the client to explore things in their own way original to Clean Language. Other approaches to therapy, whether talking therapies or kinds that involve body or energy work, do that too. And it isn't just the care you take to work with the client's exact words – other therapists were doing that before Clean Language came along. But when you combine all three of these things, something interesting starts to happen. What makes Clean Language so effective a tool in mind/body awareness is this: the questions are specifically devised to focus on the simplest elements of human experience – directly through the senses and in the moment, rather than indirectly through the many layers of abstraction that the thinking mind constructs. In the words of Basil Panzer, David Grove's co-author of *Resolving Traumatic Memories* (1989, p.xi), 'The therapist's clean language facilitates a state of purposeful, focused, uncontaminated self-absorption.' And what does that do?

THE BODY'S SENSE OF THE BRAIN

The most practical answer is that it means you are talking a language that the body understands. The body thinks, but it doesn't think in words. Imagine being your own body for a minute. What would that be like? Up there is a head that thinks incessantly, eyes and ears that are constantly monitoring the sights and sounds of the outside world, and a brain that is preoccupied so much of the time with responding to or planning how to act in or influence that world. The body's senses of touch, taste, smell and movement offer a more direct connection between the world beyond the skin and the internal one, but in the hierarchy of the senses, these are all considered by the head up there to have much lower status than seeing and hearing. From the body's point of view, the head lives in an audio-visual virtual reality, in front of a computer screen or a television for most of the day. For the body, the basic units of information are not words or images, but much simpler elements of experience which are most of the time beyond awareness – the shape, colour, size, movement, texture, feel, location, smell and sound of things. Understanding how we process information in the body means being willing to work with smaller, simpler chunks of information – ones which may be confusing or frustrating for the everyday mind, which is used to labelling things rapidly and moving on.

Imagine two people in an art gallery. A young man is walking slowly from picture to picture, taking time to notice what kind of response he has to each. Meanwhile, a woman holding a notebook is walking rapidly from room to room, looking only briefly at each picture before making a note and moving briskly on. The young man is a visitor to the gallery, entranced to see these great paintings, and in an open state of mind, musing, absorbed and responsive. The woman works at the gallery and is busy planning a new exhibition. She has seen these pictures many times before and has no time right now to look at them more deeply. Her state is the one we are usually in as we get on with the business of the day – it enables us to get things done, but the young man's state is the one you need to be in to communicate with your body.

So Clean questions bring the mind back to a state of pure perception – they reawaken the ability to experience things in a more childlike way, with openness and curiosity. In the way a toddler explores the external world, sometimes with delight, sometimes with frustration, occasionally feeling helpless or scared, so Clean questions help you explore your internal world, a place which can often seem just as strange a mixture of the delightful and the difficult. As the practitioner learning how to guide your client step by step, remember that basic parental skill of knowing when to leave a child to explore things on their own while staying close at hand in case they need you. How Clean questions help us to connect with and make sense of this internal world is the subject of the next chapter as we look at the full set of Clean questions, and exactly what each kind of question does.

~ 10 ~

THE 12 CORE CLEAN
LANGUAGE QUESTIONS

You've already seen how much can happen by using those first three questions. For me, one of the most elegant and impressive things about Clean Language is how much you can achieve using just those three questions alone. Another is how short the list of core Clean questions is – there are just 12 basic questions, although some have an alternative version, as you'll see. Each question is designed to focus your attention on a particular aspect of your own private landscape of reality as you experience it in the moment, and to help you make links between the different features of this landscape. Honed and perfected over many years by David Grove and his colleagues, these core questions have acquired some variations along the way depending on who is using them and the context they are being used in. I will present them here in the form that I've found most effective when you're using them in bodywork therapy.

THE CORE CLEAN QUESTIONS AND WHAT THEY DO

It's easy to forget that the way we are built as human beings predetermines how we pay attention to things and how we experience the world. In each human bodymind, a huge amount of sensory and neurological activity is constantly going on just so that we can 'make sense' of what is happening around us and within us. Of course, most of that sensing is at a completely unconscious level. In their ground-breaking book, *The Embodied Mind* (1991), a weaving-together of cognitive science with both Western and Buddhist philosophy, Francisco Varela, Evan Thompson and Eleanor Rosch proposed over 20 years ago that, 'One of the most fundamental cognitive activities that all organisms perform is categorization. By this means the uniqueness of each experience is transformed into the more limited set of learned, meaningful categories to which humans and other organisms respond' (p.176). In other words, that mass of unconscious sensory information must first be filtered into categories that the everyday mind can recognise, before we can even be aware of it.

Each Clean question is designed to direct your attention to at least one of these fundamental categories of perception. First have a look at the whole list – it's reassuring to see just how simple each question is – then we'll look in more detail at how exactly each kind of question works.

THE CORE SET OF CLEAN QUESTIONS

ATTRIBUTES
What attributes does it have, like shape, colour, texture or size?

And what kind of...X...?
And is there anything else about...X?

LOCATION
Where is it, for example inside or outside the body?

And where is...X...?

FOCUS
What draws your attention, among all the things that are competing for your attention all the time?

And what are you drawn to?

TIME AND SEQUENCE
When does it happen, and when does it happen in relation to other specific events?

And then what happens?
And what happens just before...X...?

METAPHOR
What is it like? How would you describe it in terms of something else?

And that's an...X...like what?

ORIGIN
Where does it come from? What is its source?

And where does/could...X...come from?

RELATIONSHIP
What is your relation to it and what is its relationship with other parts of your internal landscape?

And is there a relationship between...X...and...Y?

OUTCOME
What do you want to have happen, or what does something you're aware of want to have happen?

And what would you like to have happen?
And what would...X...like to have happen?

POWER
What can it do, and what can it not do?

And can...X...do...Y?

None of these questions is unique to Clean Language, but when you ask them in a Clean context, the difference starts at the level of intention – instead of gathering information to assist you in making some kind of professional judgement or diagnosis, you're simply inviting the client to take a first step into their own internal landscape, and trusting that as that landscape reveals itself, it will also reveal the clues and connections that will activate their own healing process. So now let's look in more detail at each of the core Clean questions in turn and what they're designed to do.

THE ATTRIBUTES QUESTIONS

And what kind of...X...?
And is there anything else about...X?

Alternative:

And does...X...have a size, shape, colour, direction, age, etc.?

Our attention is constantly shifting and one reason why the body creates symptoms is to have a way of repeatedly bringing us back to a problem it wants us to pay attention to. These very simple opening questions help that process, by encouraging a client to stay focused on a particular issue and to get more curious about how they are actually experiencing it right now. Whether the client is talking about a symptom (something they don't want), or an outcome (something they do want), you become more and more aware that the words themselves are only labels, so these questions are also a reminder to you, the practitioner, not to assume that you know what any particular words your client uses actually mean, and not to assume that the client knows either.

Asking '**And what kind of…?**' is an invitation to notice the attributes and characteristics of whatever that label stands for: not only things like size, shape, colour, texture and movement, but also less tangible but equally important qualities to do with mood, behaviour, attitudes and beliefs.

For example, say the client is a hard-working professional in his 40s who says, 'I want to feel more balanced.' Since feeling balanced is usually considered a good thing in bodywork therapy, as the practitioner I might feel tempted to nod in agreement, start looking for diagnostic information about his sense of imbalance, and wonder how I might go about helping him feel more balanced. It's at this point that you realise how fundamentally different the Clean Language approach really is. Since the basic assumption behind all the Clean questions is that the client knows far more about their problem – and far more about its solution – than they think they do, your real aim is to accompany them in a process of self-inquiry. To start this process, you just begin exploring the attributes of 'balance' with the simplest and most multi-purpose tool you have at your disposal, the '**And what kind of…?**' question.

 – I want to feel more balanced.

And what kind of more balanced?

Most clients will never have paid much attention to what lies beyond that conceptual label 'balance', and it is always fascinating to watch this internal inquiry begin, as they sense within themselves that there is indeed some kind of answer to it – an answer making its way into consciousness, through subtle bodily shifts, eye movements, tilting of the head and so on. We've already seen some powerful examples of how this apparently obvious question, when used with Clean intentions, can open the way to real insight. Eventually, the client says:

 – I just want…uh…(he looks up, then to the right, then forwards, while shifting his weight from one buttock to the other)…

I suppose more of a balance between what I *want* to do and all the stuff I *have* to do.

The answer may not have come as a shape or a colour or a size, but it develops the abstract label of 'balance' into something tangible (the shifting of weight is a sign that the bodymind is contributing to the dialogue) and something about balance between two different things. This is where the second Attributes question is so useful: '**And is there anything else about...X...?**' Making no assumptions, (except the fundamental Clean Language assumption that there may be more to discover about these keywords), it keeps the space open for the client to go further if he wants to, and offers the practitioner a very handy way to encourage that exploration. For the practitioner, this question is also a kind of windscreen wiper for the mind, wiping it clear – at least for a moment – of all those personal thoughts, suggestions and lines of inquiry that keep popping into it in response to what your client has just said. So back to the example above:

The client has just said he wants, 'more of a balance between what I *want* to do and all the stuff I *have* to do.'

And is there anything else about more of a balance between what you want to do and all the stuff you have to do?
- Euh...it's like all the stuff I want to do gets squashed by everything I have to do.

The keyword 'squashed' here, with its very kinaesthetic quality, is a perfect invitation to ask the next kind of Clean question, one you already know; perhaps the most under-used of all the core Clean questions but one of the most effective at getting information to start flowing between the everyday mind and the bodymind, the simple question of '**Where...?**'.

THE LOCATION QUESTION

And where is...X...?

Alternatives:

And where exactly is...X...?
And whereabouts is...X...?
If your hand could go to...X..., where would it go?

Metaphors can easily sound like abstract constructions, existing nowhere but in the imagination. The **'Where...?'** questions are a very effective way of giving these metaphors a sudden and surprising reality by showing that they are indeed located somewhere in relation to the client's body. All you have to do is to ask, **'And where...?'** In this case, the implicit metaphor 'squashed' is the obvious keyword for the next question.

And when the stuff you want to do gets squashed by everything you have to do, where is squashed?
 – Where? Uh...(looking up and then down at the floor)...well, I suppose it's around here (indicating solar plexus/diaphragm area with his right hand).

Notice that the client's answer to the **'And where...?'** question came as a gesture, as well as in words ('around here'). This little moment is always worth celebrating, as the **'Where...?'** question helps the client discover that they know something about this at a bodymind level. To acknowledge this, just adapt your next Clean question accordingly, pointing to wherever in their own body they gestured towards. We will come back to this client later in the chapter when we look at the Relationship questions.

WHY 'WHERE...?' IS SO IMPORTANT
Why is **'Where...?'** so important, this sense of where we are in relation to things and where they are in relation to us? At the simple level of safety, we want to be as far away as possible from any potential threat, and this basic animal level of risk assessment underlies our sensory processing in every waking moment. At the other end of the scale of attachment, when we love something, we want it to be close. In a TV documentary I once saw a mother

talking about what she went through after losing both her young children to a rare and incurable illness. 'It felt like I had been dropped into the middle of a vast empty space. I didn't know where they were.' Before she said anything about her thoughts or emotions, the first thing she mentioned was this simple sense of 'Where...? Where are they?' For me, this was the most poignant possible reminder of how fundamental location in space is to our sense of attachment.

The '**Where...?**' question is obviously one you'd normally ask about any physical symptom as you take a history. But when you use it in a Clean context, you're also encouraging information to start flowing between mind and body. To take an example from my own meridian-based kind of bodywork, a client will often give me an unconscious non-verbal signal, say by running a finger directly along an acupuncture channel on the front of their thigh, before they have even told me that what has brought them to see me is a problem with their knee. As the practitioner, I know which part of the knee that meridian goes through, and what mental, emotional and even spiritual associations it may have. It is as if their bodymind is trying to communicate directly with me in its own kind of sign language. When you use the '**Where...?**' questions, you help the client connect with the symptom in a conscious, cognitive way.

If you follow up your first '**And where is...?**' question with '**And whereabouts is...?**' or '**And where exactly is...?**' you are inviting your client to focus more attention on this troubled spot, and in a more precise way. Often this alone is enough for them to be able to start connecting with what their body is trying to tell them, to feel something that they weren't feeling before. Clean questions can help to translate this response into an image, a metaphor or a key phrase that the conscious mind can then make sense of.

Although the '**Where...?**' questions make intuitive sense when you ask them about physical problems, they can also be very revealing even when the issue is not obviously located in the body at all. This is because we are so deeply programmed as humans to notice the location of things, and especially where things are in relation to our own bodies, that we tend unconsciously to ascribe a location to everything, no matter how abstract and no matter whether it's inside our own head or body, or outside us. Your client may give you a funny look if they are talking about wanting more recognition at work and you ask, '**And where is** more recognition?' But if you just stay silent, they may be surprised to find that there's an answer. For example, in *The Five Minute Coach*, by Lynne Cooper and Mariette Castellino, which is about using Clean Language in a business coaching context, the client starts by saying he wants to focus on 'Prioritising'. After a few Clean questions, his coach asks him, '**And where is** prioritising?'

> Chris: I'm not sure...actually it's in front of me.
>
> Coach: And when it's in front of you, whereabouts in front of you?
>
> Chris: Just here (*Chris gestures to a space from left to right of his body, at waist level*).
>
> Coach: And it's there (*pointing to space Chris has just indicated*). Given what you now know, what would you like to have happen?
>
> Chris: I'd like to find it easy to meet my deadlines.
>
> (Cooper and Castellino 2012, p.77)

From the bodymind point of view, what's interesting about this is that, although Chris may not realise it, the '**Where...?**' and '**Whereabouts...?**' questions have already given his outcome a location in relation to his own body, and developed it from the abstract 'Prioritising' to something that has, in the word 'easy', a bit more of a felt sense to it: 'To find it easy to meet my deadlines'.

To the everyday mind, it makes little sense to ask, '**And where is...?**' about a problem or outcome that sounds abstract or diffuse, like 'Depressed' or 'Standing up to my boss'. If your client looks blank when you do ask this, you can always get the bodymind to help by asking, '**If your hand could show you where "depressed" is, where would it go?**' When you ask Location questions about the things that matter most to your client, you almost always find they bring information into awareness which comes from and encourages communication between body and mind.

THE FOCUS QUESTION

And what are you drawn to?

Alternative:

And when X and Y (...and Z), what are you drawn to most?

If, as you talk to your client, various issues come up, it may not be obvious where to start. The Focus question is important reminder to you as a Clean practitioner that it's not your decision to make. You will probably already have your own intuitions about where you want to begin, but asking this question is a very important part of the Clean approach because it engages the client in that decision. Notice the phrase 'drawn to' is designed to appeal to the client's whole mind/body sense of where to start. For example, if you ask, 'Which of those issues do you *think* is most important?' it suggests a much more cerebral kind of answer, as if your client has a mental to-do list or is simply asking, 'Which problem do I want to get rid of first?' Exploring the issues with a few Clean questions invites the client to respond in a more mindful way and to be more open to what the body knows about how apparently separate issues may in some way be connected.

Another way to use the Focus question is when, if you're exploring the client's outcome, they find other, maybe bigger or better outcomes starting to appear. Say, for example, a young man has chronic wrist pain which is interfering with his work. As you ask Clean questions about it, more and more information comes into awareness, and the question of what to focus on becomes more complicated. His first outcome may be:

- I just want my wrist to be back to normal.

And what kind of back to normal?
- Looser and freer.

And is there anything else about looser and freer?
- Then I can get on with everything I have to do a lot more easily.

And is there anything else about getting on with everything you have to do a lot more easily?
- (Sighing) Well, for a start, I'd feel a lot more relaxed about work.

And is there anything else about feeling a lot more relaxed about work?
- I'd feel stronger.

And where is stronger?
- Here (puts hand on chest).

And is there anything else about there?
- (Sighing again) It's all been making me so irritable and snappy.

At this point, a lot of things have come up. As the practitioner, all you have to do is summarise (which is a lot easier if you've been taking notes of keywords and gestures) and ask the Focus question:

And when you want your wrist to feel looser and freer, and you can get on with everything you have to do a lot more easily, and you feel more relaxed about work, and you feel stronger there (indicating client's chest), **what are you drawn to most?**
- Feeling stronger (putting hand back on chest).

This gives you an outcome ('Feeling stronger') you can confidently focus on, because the client has verbally and somatically confirmed that there seems to be something especially important about it. You can still come back to ask about other aspects of his outcome, but now you know that the decision about what to focus on first is his, not yours.

One more way to use this Focus question is as a kind of mindfulness exercise to help the transition between asking Clean questions and beginning the bodywork treatment. Once you have discussed all the issues with your client, you can ask them to sit back or lie down, let things settle and just stay with their breathing for a couple of minutes. Then summarise the list of keywords you have noted down and ask, '**And when you** take some time like this, of all those things, **what you are drawn to most?**' Don't be surprised if their bodymind draws their attention to something different from anything they've mentioned before. Just accept what is offered and find a way to use that as a starting point for the treatment, perhaps using the Clean Touch process described in Chapter 31.

THE TIME AND SEQUENCE QUESTIONS

And when...X...then what happens?
And what happens next?

Alternatives:

And what happens just before...X...?
And what happens just after...X...?

Space and time are where life happens, so questions about '**When...?**' make just as much intuitive sense to most clients as questions about '**Where...?**' And in the same way, when you ask them with Clean intentions, they can take you to surprising places.

Time questions are not just about clock time. They can be really useful in unravelling the *sequence* of events that underlies a problem behaviour or a healing process. The first two, '**And when...X...then what happens?**' and '**And what happens next?**' are interchangeable and can be used to explore either a problem or an outcome. For example, a woman in her early 40s comes to you with hip pain. She says she used to love running but gave it up when pregnant with her first child. Now she has taken it up again because her team at work is doing a charity fundraising run.

– When I'm running, after a while I get an ache here in my hip.

And when *you get an ache there in your hip,* ***then what happens?***
- If I keep running, it just gets worse, so I have to stop; it's really annoying.

As far as the physical problem goes, she feels the pain, it gets worse, and then she has to stop, and that's the end of the sequence of events. But is it? Let's see what happens if you ask the same question one more time, with this new information.

And *you have to stop and it's really annoying, and* ***then what happens?***
- I start to panic because I'm training for a charity run. My whole team at work is doing it and I've got a lot of sponsors who've pledged money.

Shall we risk asking one more Clean question, using 'panic' as the next keyword?

And *you start to panic, and* ***then what happens?***
- Then I start thinking about how awful it would be if my hip gives out and I let everyone down.

And when *you start thinking about how awful it would be if your hip gives out and you let everybody down,* ***then what happens?***
- Actually, I can feel a bit of a twinge there. That's odd; I don't usually feel it until I've been running for a while.

Already, we have moved from a hip problem to an issue involving panic and letting people down. You often find, as you use Clean questions to help a client focus on their symptom, that they start becoming aware of it in the moment. She's just discovered that she can feel it even though she's not actually running, just talking about running. For many people this can be quite a discovery, and evidence that there really is such a thing as mind/body communication. She came in thinking that the problem with her hip was purely physical and now she's beginning to realise that her concern about letting people down may also be involved.

Of course, it's common enough that worrying about a physical problem can in itself make that problem worse, but it wouldn't be very Clean to assume that this is all that's going on. For example, later in the session a long-forgotten incident from her early running days might re-emerge, in which she pushed herself too hard for fear of letting teammates down, and suffered an injury because of it. The body remembers these things. In that case, there's another Time and Sequence question you can use to help release an embedded neuro-muscular memory, and that's, '**And what happens just before…?**'

FRAME BY FRAME

The '**Just before…**' and '**Just after…**' questions allow you to look in much closer detail at what happens moment by moment in any particular sequence of behaviour, bringing a frame-by-frame precision that can unlock unconscious parts of that sequence. For example, say your client is a man in his late 20s in a corporate job who has been getting panic attacks when giving presentations to large groups. He has already told you that his outcome is 'To be able to trust myself to stay calm and focused when I talk to large groups'. Then you start to explore the sequence of symptoms:

So what happens first when you get a panic attack?
- I'm not sure what the first thing is, but there's a kind of pressure around me, and I start sweating a lot, and there's a bit of a hollow sound in my ears and sometimes I even feel as if I'm going to faint.

Since we're exploring a sequence of events, let's focus on the very first one he mentioned.

And what happens just before there's a kind of pressure around you?
- Nothing. It just comes out of the blue. In fact, the last time it happened, I was just thinking, 'That's good, I'm not getting any panicky feelings', and – boom! – it started.

That 'Nothing' indicates that something in this sequence is out of the client's conscious awareness. So, again, we ask the '**Just before…**' question about the first thing he *is* aware of:

And what happens just before boom!?
- (Closing eyes and tilting head down) There's a kind of edge...

What kind of edge?
- Like a precipice.

And when there's a kind of edge, like a precipice, is there anything else about that edge, like a precipice?
- It's like it's just a dark black abyss.

And what happens just before there's a kind of edge, like a dark black abyss?

Here the therapist is using the '**Just before...?**' question as a kind of safety rope, bringing the client back from the edge. It's as if you are running the film backwards in slow motion.

- It's like I'm holding on to the side of a mountain, on a very narrow path, and the rock is very black and slippery.

And is there anything else about that very narrow and slippery path?
- It's like it's so narrow and slippery I can't help thinking about falling off.

And what happens just before you can't help thinking about falling off?
- (A pause, and his expression changes from anxiety to one of focused concentration) Before that it's like I'm sure-footed, even though the path isn't any wider, and my weight is even on both feet.

And when your weight is even on both feet, then what happens?
- Then I can do it...(laughing)...and there's a great view from up here!

And when you can do it, and there's a great view, then what happens?

Having pulled back to a place of safety, the practitioner now uses the '**And then what happens?**' question to invite the client to move forward in this new direction.

- It's like I'm on a tightrope. I did that once in a team-building exercise and it was fun. I had to hold the balancing pole in both hands to steady me, and to go slowly, step by step.

Now the client has spontaneously remembered an experience from the past which is both relevant and resourceful, so it's important to include that in the next question.

And when *you hold the balancing pole in both hands, and you go slowly, step by step,* **then what happens?**
- I feel very centred. It feels good.

And is there anything else about *very centred?*
- No…I'm just me.

And when *you're just you,* **then what happens?**
- Then everyone watching me is just who *they* are.

And when *you're just you, and everyone watching you is just who they are,* **what happens** *to that pressure around you?*

This is an example of the Relationship question, which we will be looking at soon. Here it's used to check how the original problem of 'pressure' may have already changed.

- It might still be there, but I realise now it's coming from me, not from them.

And when *you realise it's coming from you and not from them,* **what would you like to have happen?**

This is the Outcome question, one of the most important questions in the whole Clean approach.

- For it not to be there at all!

And when *it's not there at all,* **then what happens?**
- Oh! That's scary – I'm wobbling again, as if I'm going to fall.

The client's desire – for the problem to 'not to be there at all' – seems to have produced an odd reaction from his bodymind. If his panic attacks disappeared completely it would be 'scary'. The bodymind often communicates in this kind of way; all you need to do is ask another '**Just before...?**' question:

And what happens just before it's scary and you're wobbling again?
- It's like I need some of that pressure to hold me up, but it needs to be more around my body, not around my head.

*And when it's more around your body, and not around your head, and you're presenting to a large group, **then what happens?***
- I'm fine; it supports me and it protects me, and even if I'm nervous I can still feel quite excited, instead of just dreading it.

In this example, the practitioner uses the '**Just before...**' and '**Just after...**' questions at the start to help the client discover a vivid metaphor for the panic attacks. Then towards the end, the '**Just before**' and '**Then what happens?**' questions help him realise that the 'pressure' is not the problem in itself; it's more about where and how much pressure he needs. This would be a very interesting place to begin a treatment from, and as you work directly with the body through movement, or touch, ask more Clean questions as you go. When you finish, you can ask again about the metaphor of pressure that he started out with, to see how it is different now.

THE METAPHOR QUESTION

And that's an...X...like what?

Alternative:

And what is...X...like?

These questions are designed to encourage the client to find a metaphor for what they're talking about, rather than simply telling you the story of what happened to them, or talking about it in purely abstract or sensory terms. We have already seen how metaphors are an essential part of the way we communicate with ourselves and each other. 'A pain in the neck', 'hard to swallow', 'light-hearted', 'spaced out', 'full of beans' or 'hard-boiled' are all metaphors – ways of thinking about one thing in terms of another, and a natural product of the mind's insatiable desire to associate separate experiences which seem to have similar qualities.

Everyone has their own personal set of metaphors for the most important things in life, and indeed for life itself. For Sally Bowles life is a cabaret; for other people life may be a battle, a game, a journey or…well, what is it for you? In fact, these metaphors are a kind of code, or software program, which play a powerful role in how we interpret and respond to what is going on around us and within us.

As we saw in Chapter 8, metaphors are a hugely important part of how the bodymind communicates with the everyday mind. But while some clients will present you almost immediately with a metaphorical description of what ails them, or what they want, many clients tend to keep their metaphors more hidden and prefer to communicate in abstract or matter-of-fact language. The Metaphor questions are designed to help people take that extra step into a more associative, creative way of thinking, connecting the left brain to the right brain, and the mind to the body. The Clean question for this is '**And that's an…X…like what?**' The normal conversational version of this would be, '**And what is…X…like?**' Sometimes that will be enough of an invitation to elicit a metaphor from your client, but putting '**like what?**' at the end of the question is designed to make that invitation more emphatic, since the last words of any sentence are the ones that tend to be remembered most easily and to have the most effect.

However you ask it, you often have to work a little before your client comes up with a metaphor. In the following example, the practitioner's first '**What's that like?**' question doesn't produce a metaphor. The client, a woman who wants to get rid of persistent neck pain, needs more Clean questions to help her get to a point where a metaphor becomes the obvious way to define the problem. What's interesting is just how right the metaphor sounds to her when she does eventually discover it:

- I've been getting some pretty bad headaches too.

What kind of headaches?
- Almost like the migraines I had as a kid.

And where do you get those headaches?
- It usually starts over my right eye, just here, then spreads to the whole right side of my head.

And when it spreads to the whole right side of your head, **that's like what?**
- (Pauses to think) Then I notice that my breathing gets really shallow.

Even though this isn't a verbal metaphor yet, it could well be a somatic one, in which the shallow breathing is a clear signal about something not-so-clear inside. But one of my aims in using Clean questions is to help the client make some sense of their somatic experience, so when something like this happens, I just carry on, waiting for the next opportunity to invite the client to come up with a metaphor. In this case it doesn't take long:

And when it spreads to the whole right side of your head and your breathing gets really shallow, **that's like what?**
- It's like a big steel clamp – like my head is stuck in some kind of steel clamp and I can't move. I know that sounds stupid but that's what it's like.

When your client does use a metaphor, especially a powerful one like this, remember that you don't have to know what it means. All you need to do is to carry on asking Clean questions, allowing her to explore it in more detail, and leaving it up to her to discover what the metaphor has to tell her about how to move forward with that issue.

METAPHOR AND SIMILE

One last point, in case you were wondering, *Clean Language doesn't differentiate between metaphor and simile.* Whether your client describes it with a simile ('It's *like* my head is stuck in some kind of steel clamp') or a metaphor ('My head *is* stuck in some kind of steel clamp'), one thing is being described in terms of another, and so in Clean Language we treat them both as metaphors. But sometimes you may notice a difference in 'charge' between the two: that is, a difference in how much energy is invested in the pattern that's being described. Simile *invites* you to make the connection by using the word 'like', while metaphor is more manipulative – it presents the comparison as if it were a fact. Dropping the 'like' gives a metaphor directness and impact, as you might notice if you say slowly out loud to yourself 'My love is *like* a red, red rose', and then 'My love *is* a red, red rose'. For me there is a distinctly different sensation inside my head, as if to make sense of the metaphor, my brain has to shift up a gear.

THE ORIGIN QUESTION

And where does/could...X...come from?

This question about the source or origin of something can bring up several different kinds of answer, but one of the most obvious is to take the client back into the past. In this way you could say that it is simply another version of the questions about location and time: where and when does that (keyword) come from? And of course, it's a question common to many different kinds of approach, whether it be bodywork, energy psychology or talking therapy – seeking the origin of the problem so that it can be acknowledged, aligned, balanced, somatically released, analysed, deconstructed, accepted, loved, forgiven or dispatched into a parallel universe – whatever technique you use in your particular kind of therapy.

But there can be other kinds of answer to the question of where something comes from. A thing can come from a place, a person, a process, a culture, a relationship or a behaviour, or even (in some cases) the future, as well as from the past. For example, when you ask a client about where their chronic back pain could have come from, if they say, 'I've had it since my early teens,' they're obviously talking about the past. But they might say, 'My dad had the same thing,' so they might be implying that the source is a person. Or, 'I think it has something to do with the way I sit'; in this case it has to do with a behaviour. If they say, 'I got it from a cycling accident when I got concussion,' they may be thinking of the actual trauma of 'concussion' as the source. And if your client says, 'It's just bad karma, I guess,' don't panic; all you have to do is ask, '**And is there anything else about** bad karma?' and see what happens next.

THE RELATIONSHIP QUESTION

And is there a relationship between...X...and...Y?

Alternative:

And when...X...what happens to...Y?

You may wonder if relationships can be considered one of the simplest elements of perception, since relationships are by definition a more complex class of experience than things like size or shape or location. But relationships are certainly one of the most *fundamental* aspects of perception. Before we are born we are already in a relationship with the movements, moods and sounds of our mother's bodymind; in fact perception itself depends on the relationship between perceiver and perceived. So looking for the relationships between the things that come up in response to Clean questions is an essential part of the process, especially since Clean questions are such a powerful way of exploring one of the defining relationships of being human – the relationship between body and mind.

You can ask the Relationship question about any two aspects of a client's experience that you are curious about. When you ask this question and there is a relationship, say between a physical sensation and a difficult memory, the response can be slow and subtle, as if the bodymind is testing how much it can trust you, or it may be immediate and powerful, like the moment when you 'get' a joke. If the relationship is tenuous or undeveloped, it may take the client some time even to acknowledge that it's there or to get a sense of it. Remember to ask this question in the spirit of Clean Language and not to assume that there has to be a relationship between the things you're asking about, at least not one that seems significant to your client.

A simple and very effective way to use the Relationship question is to wait until you notice your client experiencing some real shift in response to your Clean questions, and listen for what keywords or gestures (Y) accompany that shift. Then track back to the beginning of the conversation and remember the keyword (X) your client used to describe their initial problem or outcome. Now you are ready to ask, **'And is there a relationship between (Y) and (X)?'** For example, let's come back to our client in the Attributes section of this chapter who wanted, 'more of a balance between what I *want* to do and all the stuff I *have* to do'. The last thing he said was, 'It's like all the stuff I want to do gets squashed by everything I have to do.'

And where is *squashed?*
- How do you mean, where?

If your hand could show you where *squashed* **is, where would it go?**

This is a useful suggestion to help clients move from a logical-mind response into a bodymind response.

- Around there.

As he says this, he raises his arms, palms facing each other in front of his chest. He is silent for a few breaths as his arms seem to adjust themselves into a posture of balanced equilibrium. Now you're ready to ask the Relationship question:

And is there a relationship between how your arms are now, **and** having more of a balance between what you want to do and all the stuff you have to do?

- I don't know. (As he says this, you notice he takes a deeper breath, then his left shoulder relaxes and his jaw muscles soften.)

What just happened?

This is a very useful question to ask whenever you want your client to notice that something has changed.

- I'm not sure, but it feels different now.

What kind of different?

- More peaceful here (touching the centre of his chest and letting his hands drop down into his lap).

In this example, the Relationship question connected the equilibrium of the client's posture to his original outcome of having more balance, and it has produced the positive result of feeling 'more peaceful' in the chest. This could be useful diagnostic information and a good place to ask him if he'd like to start the bodywork-part treatment.

You can also use the Relationship question to connect a resource that emerges during the mind/body treatment that you do, with the client's original problem or outcome. Once the client has experienced the full benefit of an acupuncture treatment, a CranioSacral session, an Alexander lesson or whatever it may be, they will almost certainly be in a wiser and more open state than when they came in. The keywords they use to describe this state will probably be quite generic ones like 'lighter', 'more grounded', 'more at peace with myself' and so on. Just put these keywords into the Relationship question to remind them of their original outcome and consciously connect this new resource to it. For example:

And how are you now?

- Mmm…well…definitely different. (Clients often find it hard to answer this question immediately after a treatment because the verbal mind may have been having a rest and is just waking up again.) It's as though there's more of me.

*And when there's more of you, **is there a relationship between** more of you and having more balance between what you want to do **and** all the things you have to do?*

- (After a long pause with eyes closed) Yes, I don't feel so guilty about doing what I want to do.

*And when you don't feel so guilty about doing what you want to do, **what happens to** all the things you have to do?*

- They get done, or they don't. Or someone else can do them. I don't know. It's not so important. (Smiling) That sounds terrible, doesn't it?

It's the end of the session and, as sometimes happens, the client is discovering a whole new aspect to the issue – guilt about doing what he wants to do. For now, as far as keeping it Clean goes, a gentle reminder that your time is up, preferably said with a smile, would be:

*And when they get done, or they don't, or someone else can do them and it's not so important, and that sounds terrible, **is that an okay place to finish for now?***

For most clients, the answer will be 'Yes', but if for any reason your client says 'No', and needs to talk some more, then in my opinion, it's best to keep any further talk free of Clean Language. Clean questions open things up, so don't ask any more when you want to close a session; just identify the problem, suggest some 'homework' if appropriate, and agree a date for your next appointment.

THE OUTCOME QUESTIONS

And what would you like to have happen?
And what would…X…like to have happen?

Follow-up questions:

And what needs to happen for…(outcome)?
And what else needs to happen for…(outcome)?

We will be looking at the Outcome questions in more detail in the following two chapters. They get two chapters to themselves because they are some of the most important of all the Clean questions, and a foundation of the whole Clean approach.

No doubt you already ask your clients some kind of question about what they want to achieve from their work with you. And you've probably noticed how some clients find it easy to answer, others struggle and still others have no idea what you're talking about. For the moment, just notice what happens when you use the outcome question and follow it up with one or two more Clean questions. If it works for them, this can create a powerful shift in the way clients approach a session and what they expect to get out of it. The power, as well as the challenge, of using the Outcome questions is that they appeal directly to the client's sense of 'agency'; by asking them what they want, you remind them that they're not just observing their own experience – they can bring choice, intention and willpower to their situation too. For some clients this is liberating; for others it may seem scary or simply unrealistic.

For example, imagine a man in his late 60s who has recently retired. He has come with 'A vague kind of stiff neck feeling', and after a few questions also mentions finding it 'Hard to stay focused'. You ask your first Outcome question:

And when it's hard to stay focused and you have that vague kind of stiff neck feeling, **what would you like to have happen?**
– Just to feel looser in my neck – I think that's what I really need.

And if you could feel looser *in your neck,* **where is** looser *in your neck?*

Notice 'if you could' is used here as a more invitational form of 'And when...?'

- Um, round the back, at the top of the spine, I think.

And where exactly round the back at the top of the spine?
- Here (he puts the palm of his hand around the back of his neck and lets his head drop forwards, stretching the back of the neck).

And is there anything else about there where your hand is?
- It's starting to relax a bit, actually. That's funny...(speaking more slowly)...like a weight's being lifted off.

At a moment like this, when the client is allowing himself some felt communication with his own body, you can be pretty sure that at some internal level he is getting a more vivid or detailed sense of his original outcome, and to check that, it's good to ask the Outcome question again.

(Speaking at the same slower pace as the client) **And when** it's like a weight's being lifted off, **what else needs to happen** to feel looser in your neck?
- I'd like my head to be beautifully poised on the top of my neck, and to feel really solid down here (putting his hand on his abdomen).

Notice how this second use of the Outcome questions evokes a very different kind of response. From 'Just to feel looser in my neck,' we've moved to an aesthetic sense of poise in the head and neck, and a connection to the centre of gravity in the belly, where he probably feels this poise comes from.

And when your head is beautifully poised on top of your neck, and you feel really solid down there, **then what happens?**
- (Slowly letting head come upright) Then I feel a lot more focused.

And is there anything else about a lot more focused?
- (Frowning) Yeah, that's when I get this awful 'retired' feeling of having nothing to do, and I get this 'euchh' (slumping in chest, and tightening up again round the neck).

Ah! Just when you seemed to be getting somewhere, the client slips back into the same pattern he started the session with. But here the practitioner simply accepts what is offered and notices how the new piece of behaviour – the slump in the chest and the feeling of having nothing to do – contributes to the tightening of the neck muscles. You could go on exploring this stuck state with all the other kinds of Clean question, but let's see what happens if you use an Outcome question again:

And when there's that awful 'retired' feeling of having nothing to do and you get this 'euchh' like that (indicating the client's slumping chest), **what would you like to have happen?**
- Space to breathe.

And is there anything else about space to breathe?
- (Sitting up straighter, and expanding his chest more as he breathes in) It's not so bad.

And when it's not so bad, and you sit up straighter like that, and there's space to breathe, **then what happens to the 'euchh'?**

Notice that as well as repeating the client's words, the practitioner puts his non-verbal response into the question ('Sit up straighter like that'), helping him to be more aware that his body has been making its own contribution to the dialogue.

- It isn't so strong; in fact it just goes.

And would that be a good place to start exploring this with some bodywork?

In this example the practitioner used an Outcome question three times: first to elicit an initial outcome ('to feel looser in my neck'), then to enrich and add to that first outcome ('my head to be beautifully poised on the top of my neck, and to feel really solid down here') and then to help the client find what he needs to do to avoid getting stuck in his familiar problematic pattern ('space to breathe' – which may have metaphorical meanings for him).

Remember that, however many times you ask the Outcome question, you can then use other Clean questions to enhance the client's sense of that outcome. For example, simply by asking, '**And what happens next?**' a few times, you can help a client turn their initial outcome from something that may sound tentative or unconvincing (for example, there may be an 'If only...' quality to the way they say it) into something more vivid and compelling. The client is immediately offered the opportunity to go beyond the loop of mental dialogue that they may be repeating to themselves day after day, to starting to think about what they really want. Asking, '**And then what happens?**' or '**And is there anything else about...?**' can lift the client's sense of the outcome to another level by exploring just what achieving this outcome would mean to them.

On the other hand, if there is still something tentative or unconvincing in how they talk about their outcome, that note of doubt is important to acknowledge. Sometimes asking '**And then what happens...?**' repeatedly about the outcome can seem like pumping up a balloon too far, until it's about to burst. Make sure you check for any reservations or resistance. Which brings us to the final category in the core set of Clean questions.

THE POWER QUESTION

And can/could...X...do Y?

The Power question can be used as a kind of reality check if your client seems too positive or too negative, too fearful or too enthusiastic, in the way they are answering your questions. For example, let's come back to the young man who was having panic attacks when presenting to large groups. The first thing he was aware of about those attacks was a sense of pressure. With the help of a few Clean questions, his metaphor transformed from precipice to tightrope, and he realised that this pressure was coming from him, not from the people in the group.

And when** you realise it's coming from you and not from them, **what would you like to have happen?
 - For it not to be there at all!

This is classic wishful thinking, and transfers the 'pressure' to the therapist, who may well be wondering how to respond Cleanly when the client's outcome seems unrealistic or even counter-productive in the context of the work they've done so far. A simple response is to ask:

***And can** it not be there at all?*
 - (After a long pause with eyes closed) I don't think so. I was trying to visualise it going away, but it won't all go.

Sometimes clients do this. In response to a Clean question, they try some other therapeutic technique they already know like visualisation or positive thinking, whether it fits with the Clean approach or not. That's okay. At least he's found out in his own way that the symptom of pressure is not going to disappear. With another question or two, you can easily help him to the same realisation that he had in the earlier example, that it's not the pressure itself, but how much of it that is the real issue.

Another way to use the Power question is to double-check what a client has achieved during the session. For example, here, with the same client, the Power question is used with another version of the Outcome question – '**And what needs to happen…?**' – to help the client come up with a practical plan of action:

 - It's like I need some of that pressure to hold me up, but it needs to be more around my body, not around my head.

***And can** it be more around your body and not around your head?*
 - Yes, then it supports me and it protects me.

And what needs to happen, for it to be more around your body and not around your head?

- I need to remember that tightrope, and holding the balance pole in both hands!

And how can you remember that?

- Like this (he holds his two hands down just in front of his thighs, fingers slightly curved as if holding the balance pole, eyes half closed and focusing on his breathing, creating a physiological anchor which can remind him of his new strategy). Just taking some time to be alone before a meeting to stand like this and breathe like this and remember to just be me.

HOW CLEAN SHOULD I BE?

That is the core set of 12 Clean questions, plus a few useful alternatives, but of course there are others. In his radical and liberating book about Clean Language, *Trust Me, I'm the Patient* (2012) psychotherapist Philip Harland lists 40 Clean questions, and there are many situations where you might want to make up your own or use a less strictly Clean, more conversational style. Sometimes I just ask, 'How do you mean…?' and add the client's keywords. Sometimes a modified Clean question pops into my head that I know intuitively will be the right one for that particular client. David Grove liked to allow himself time to 'muse' during his Clean dialogues with clients, working from the principles that *make* a question Clean as much as from the standard list.

But please remember, as you start to experiment, that there is a world of difference between finding the perfect Clean way of asking a particular client a particular question, and slipping back into your own personal conversational habits. Almost invariably, this is what people do as they start learning Clean Language. Old habits keep re-presenting themselves, the therapist's mind becomes full of suggestions about how to ask a better question than the Clean version, therapeutic notions flood in about what would really be more useful to say next, and with them come your own probably quite unconscious preferences and personal judgements. Clean Language makes enormous demands on your ability to keep all of this out of the client's space, but at the same time provides you with the perfect tools to do so. David Grove said that Clean questions allow 'The I-ness of the therapist…to cease to exist' (Grove and Panzer 1989, p.103). This is a high aim indeed, but one that is worth keeping in mind even on the beginner's slopes of Clean. How you manage this balance between using more conversational language and knowing when to ask a Clean question will vary with each person and each situation. But when in doubt, always use a Clean question first. That way you'll not only be respecting your client's space and encouraging their self-healing process, you'll also be giving yourself the practice you need to become comfortably fluent in the language of Clean.

~ 11 ~

THE CLIENT'S GOALS:
WHAT WOULD YOU LIKE
TO HAVE HAPPEN?

If you're looking for a new car or ordering food in a restaurant, you usually have some idea of what you want. Most people don't go to a car showroom just to talk about all the things that are wrong with their old car. When a waiter asks you what you'd like to order, you don't start by talking about a particular kind of food you really hated when you were eight years old. In these situations you're more focused on what you *do* want than on what you don't want. In the therapy business, of course, it's usually the other way round. We go to therapists because we have problems, we have aches and longings, holes in our energy fields, suicidal thoughts, embarrassing rashes, panic attacks, painful backs, immune systems that have turned against us, reproductive systems that won't reproduce, chakras that are spinning in the wrong direction, terminal illnesses, relationships we wish we hadn't got into but can see no way out of. And we not only have problems, we have problems about having these problems. We don't just get ill, we have negative thoughts and feelings about being ill, so that a chronic lower back pain isn't just a physical sensation but a source of irritation or embarrassment, rage or shame, anxiety or guilt; in this way our symptoms can easily become the enemy within.

WHAT YOU DON'T WANT AND WHAT YOU DO WANT

Even if you ask specifically what a client would like to get from your therapy, most people take this as an invitation to tell you more about their problem – how long they've had it, where exactly it is, how bad it can get, what might have caused it and so on. In other words, they are telling you more about what they don't want, not what they *do* want. Observing this over and over again in his clients, Moshe Feldenkrais, founder of the mind/body awareness method that bears his name, put it this way:

> Words are not used in order to express what we need or what we want. They are there like the mask we carry on our face, to hide what we want. Because most of the time we are so divorced from our feelings that we know only that kind of cerebration that connects the brain with words.[1]

Of course, taking a history is an important part of the diagnostic process, but as the word 'history' implies, it focuses the client entirely on the past rather than the future. As they talk about their problem, you may see them reconnecting with it and notice the subtle signs of how it affects them – frown lines between the eyebrows, the corners of the mouth turning down, a change in the colour in their cheeks, a slumping or tightening of the shoulders, a more aggressive or more hopeless tone of voice, or sometimes just a matter-of-fact monotone, as if they have succeeded in dissociating themselves completely from the problem. Your client is giving you a live demonstration of just how this problem is affecting them and how they are dealing with it.

---

1   Moshe Feldenkrais, transcribed from a YouTube film of him teaching, www.youtube.com/watch?v=1V_5O7KANWI

And the worse the problem, the greater the pressure you may feel to do something about it as quickly as possible. You may think it would sound more than a bit insensitive to start asking them how they would like to be or what they really want. You may be right. When a client is desperate for your help they may get quite irritable when you don't immediately jump into treatment mode. The obvious answer to 'What do you want?' is 'I want the pain to go away and to get back to normal, so please stop asking me all these questions and get on with whatever it is I'm paying you for.'

But asking your client to get clearer about what they want is very often the single most effective way you can help them, and all the other things you can do with words or touch or movement will become easier and more effective if you do. When your clients can move from being preoccupied with what is wrong with them to being curious about what would be right for them, it not only transforms the relationship they have with their symptoms, it also changes the relationship they have with themselves, with you and with what your kind of therapy can achieve for them. The problem is that just asking a client what they want is no guarantee that any of that will happen. As James Lawley, one of the most experienced Clean Language facilitators on the planet, has said, 'When you ask "What would you like to have happen?" so many clients say, "If I knew that I wouldn't be here."'[2]

The truth is that when you ask clients about the outcome they want from working with you, you're inviting them to move through up to five separate (or overlapping) stages of response. The first is simply wanting the problem to go away; the second is to think about what it would be like to get back to normal; the third is wondering if there was something about 'normal' that caused the problem in the first place; if so, the fourth is acknowledging and accepting that and finding out how to move on from that old pattern; and the fifth is finding out what it would be like to do that, to actually imagine and embody that new way of being.

---

2   James Lawley, comment at a meeting of Developing Group, London 2013.

WHAT WOULD YOU LIKE TO HAVE HAPPEN?

However you phrase it, when you ask your clients what they would like from working with you, you're asking the Outcome question. The official Clean Language version of this is, '**What would you like to have happen?**' This not only sounds quite user-friendly, it also hints in the phrase 'to have happen' that the client will be playing their own part in the process. The real aim of the Outcome question is to help your client to feel actively and responsibly engaged in the therapy rather than a passive receiver of treatment. To do this you usually need to ask it several times during the conversation, gently returning to it each time a new aspect of the problem emerges, until they can express their goal positively not just in words, but in voice and body language too.

For example, if you ask your client what they would like from the treatment, their first answer might be 'To get rid of my backache'. If they sit there with no change of expression or posture, is that really a positive answer? No. In terms of language alone, it's still focused on the negative – the client is still talking about the problem, 'backache', and their aim is to 'get rid of' it. The proof that nothing has shifted yet is that there is no change in their posture or movement. A Clean question designed to help them explore the positive sense of what they want would be, '**And what would that be like**, to get rid of your backache?' Be prepared for a blank look and a silence before the answer comes. If they've had this problem for a while, you're asking them to go to an unfamiliar place – to whatever information is in there of how their back once was, or would be, if it was strong and flexible and they were able to sit, stand or move with ease. Notice how those positive words 'strong', 'flexible' and 'move with ease' already sound very different from 'get rid of my backache'. This is because using positive words involves accessing in some way what they refer to, and that involves activating different parts of the brain from the ones they have got used to thinking with when they think about the problem in purely negative terms. This is why the answer will usually come as a shift in posture or change in breathing before it comes in words. In fact, it's through those shifts that the client first lets you know that your Outcome questions are beginning to work.

If the 'official' Outcome question sounds good to you, start using it and notice the difference it can make. If this version of the question sounds awkward to you, then experiment by asking it in different ways. Part of the art of using Clean Language is finding the words that will work for your client, and being sensitive to the subtle effects those words may have. For example, a client who looks blank when you ask, 'What would you like from this session?' with its implication that there should be one main thing they want, may find it easier to make sense of the question if you ask, 'What kind of things would you like to get from this session?' with its more open invitation to explore a range of possibilities.

Sometimes, if a client is so focused on their problem that they just don't understand what I'm asking, I use a Clean version of the well-known 'miracle question' – 'If you woke up one morning and just didn't have this problem any more, what would that be like?' Another way to do it, if they keep telling you about what they don't want, is to point this out to them. 'So if this problem, with all its symptoms that you've been telling me about, is what you don't want, what is it that you *do* want?' However you phrase the Outcome question, the key point is to keep coming back to it until their answer is in positive language and it's accompanied by a gesture or a visible shift in their energy, no matter how subtle. The Outcome question gives your client a chance to imagine and embody how they really want to be before you start your treatment. When your client starts using positive language, then in effect they have already begun their treatment. When you begin working with the techniques of your own particular therapy, you will almost certainly find that things flow more easily than if you had started by simply asking about their symptoms. Because you have explored the positive as well as the negative side of the situation, when they come to an obstacle, it won't seem like the void it might have seemed before. Now there is not just 'hope' or 'light at the end of the tunnel'; through your Clean questions they have been able to connect in an embodied way with what they really want to achieve from working with you.

A FRIEND'S BACKACHE

To give you an idea of how easily you can do this even in an informal way, here is a very simple example from a practitioner who was trying out the Outcome question for the first time.

Veena was at a friend's house; the friend had constant back pain, so she just introduced the Outcome question into their normal conversation. This is her account of what happened next:

She said her shoulders felt creaky and her back was painful, so I asked her, 'What would you really like to have happen – what would it be like if you didn't have back pain?' Observing my friend when I asked this question was amazing. She smiled and started to rock playfully backwards and forwards and side to side as she began to wonder about this possibility. Touching her back as she spoke, she said, 'I would be walking without any pain...I'd like to feel like I can walk for miles and miles and miles.' Surprised by such a positive response, I followed it up with another Clean question: 'And what is it like when you can walk for miles and miles and miles?'

My friend took a deeper breath and straightened up and her eyes began staring into the distance.

- Lots of things, my posture is good and there is lots of beauty and anticipation.

And where is the beauty and anticipation?
- In my eyes and forehead.

And is there anything else about the beauty and anticipation in *your eyes and forehead?*
- Yes, it gives me pleasure...and happiness.

When I asked her how she felt after the conversation, she said there had been a shift in her stiffness and her back and hips had loosened and were no longer painful. She also had a sense that her shoulders, though still creaky, were slowly moving downwards.

All that with only four questions, and notice how well Veena mirrored her friend's language. How would it have sounded if she'd asked, 'And what is it like when you can walk that far?' instead of 'miles and miles and miles'? There is a poetry to those repetitions which tells you that your client is responding in a creative way to the Clean questions. Just as her body began to rock, so her mind began to roll for miles and miles and miles across some imagined landscape. If you can mirror back the sounds and rhythms of that creativity as accurately as possible, you are acknowledging it, confirming it and amplifying it in a way that helps her to explore that landscape even further.

LEARNING POINTS

So before we look at some more examples of how to use the Outcome question successfully in your practice, here are three key points to remember:

1. Ask the Outcome question in a way that works for your client; in other words be sensitive to how they respond to it, and be able to adapt it so that it sounds like a realistic and inviting suggestion for each particular client, responding in their own individual way. This includes being able to back off if it seems too challenging, or asking it again if a client's first response sounds formulaic or offered just to please you.

2. Whether they answer in a negative or positive way, follow up the keywords in their answer with another Clean question; for example, 'I just want to be able to wake up in the morning without that feeling of panic.'

   And** to wake up in the morning without that feeling of panic **would be like what?

3. If necessary, return to the Outcome question two or three times until they are able to answer in positive language and something changes in their posture or the way they move.

∼ 12 ∼

WHAT HAPPENS WHEN YOU
ASK THE OUTCOME QUESTION?

The Outcome question is an invitation to your client to interrupt their usual ways of thinking about their symptoms, to listen to what their somatic mind has to tell them, and to discover how the problem itself often contains the key to the solution. As I've said, some clients find this surprisingly easy, but for others it can be a real challenge. If your client is really not responding to the Outcome question, sometimes the best approach is simply to begin the bodywork; you can always come back to it during the session or at the end, when your client will be more relaxed and more open to making sense of what their body has to tell them. Another possibility is to introduce the Outcome question gently, session by session, assessing how they respond, building up over two or three sessions to a point where they are able to answer in positive language and to feel in their body the difference that this makes. In the Interview section in Part 3, you can read about how various different bodywork therapists approach this.

There's an enormous healing potential that this question can unlock if asked in the right way and followed up with a few more

Clean questions. The more you get into the habit of asking it, the more your clients will get into the habit of asking it themselves, both in their sessions with you and in their everyday life. Some people may have spent years locked in to negative ways of thinking about a health problem only to discover that those few simple words, '**What would you like to have happen?**' are the key to opening up that healing potential.

As we've seen, most clients' first response to the Outcome question is a negative one – either an 'I don't know' or some version of 'I want the problem to go away'. If they do reply in positive language, it's usually a phrase that comes mainly from the head, from some well-thumbed mental wish list: 'to have more energy' or 'to feel calmer' or 'to have some me-time'. We are not expecting them to know consciously what they really want or need from all the things your therapy may have to offer them, but if you observe their gestures and eye movements as they reply, and follow up by asking more Clean questions, for example, 'Some me-time; what kind of me-time?', then you soon notice that it's not just the person's conscious mind but also their bodymind that's listening to you, and wanting to respond. Gestures are every bit as important as words here, because they give you vital clues to how the problem is embodied and what the outcome would really be like. Usually, these gestures are completely out of the client's awareness, as if their bodymind is trying to communicate directly with you, offering clues about what they really need.

MOVING TOWARDS THE POSITIVE

As a first example, here's a personal account by a massage therapist who was learning Clean Language while working with a professional singer.

His problem was a strange ache between the shoulder blades that had been going on for several weeks, getting more intense just before performances. After asking the usual health questions and making sure he had checked it with a doctor, the practitioner helped him to explore it with a few Clean questions. The third one produced a surprising metaphor:

And that strange ache between your shoulder blades *is like what?*
- (He stared at the floor for a few seconds and I noticed his shoulder muscles tightening) Like a flower, but with the petals closed.

And where is that flower with the petals closed?
- In a wheat field. All the wheat is about to be harvested and the flower knows it's about to be cut in two.

And where exactly is that feeling of about to be cut in two?
- (He was silent again for a minute, making micro-movements back and forth with his shoulders) All through here (he gestured towards the centre of his chest, and then outwards to his shoulders).

At this point I decided to ask the Outcome question.

And when you have that feeling all through your shoulders and chest, *what would you like to have happen?*
- I don't know. That's why I came to see you. Whatever you can do for it, I suppose.

And if whatever I can do could help, *what would you like to have happen?*
- (Another silence, a slight sigh; he raises his chin a little and I notice his shoulders drop about half a centimetre) My back and shoulders could relax.

And if your back and shoulders could relax, *what would that be like?*
- I'd like the flower to be growing somewhere safe.

During the treatment, the practitioner asked him twice what was happening in his shoulders and back, and the client felt the muscles loosening. The practitioner then took a risk by asking, '**And how is** the flower now?' – risky because it might take him right back into the sense of being about to be cut in two and make the muscles tighten again. But what actually happened was this: he suddenly took a very deep inbreath and let out a little groan, as if he was on the edge of tears. This continued for a minute, the practitioner's hand just resting on his chest, and the shoulder tension releasing significantly. Without needing another Clean question to prompt him, the client said he knew now what the tension was all about; in fact he'd known it all along – not a fear of failure exactly, but a fear of being judged, a fear of the audience not responding when he sang. By the end of the session, having made this connection, he found he could breathe much more easily into the space between his shoulder blades.

Notice what a difference it made to ask the Outcome question twice in different ways. The first one produced the classic 'I don't know' response and a desire to hand the responsibility back to the practitioner – 'Whatever you can do for it'. The second one produced a genuine somatic shift – his chin rising and his shoulders dropping a little. And the third question, 'If your back and shoulders could relax, **what would that be like?**' brings him back to the metaphor of the flower but now it has shifted to safer ground.

This example shows how it pays to insist on getting a positive response when you ask your client what they would like to have happen. It can feel like you're being a bit pushy, but for all the reasons we've already seen, the client gets a much better deal if they can put their outcome in positive language. For one thing, it changes the way the mind is affecting their body in a way they can actually feel, and it also means they are more able to make sense of any insights or emotions the treatment brings up. Notice his admission that, in some way, he'd 'known it all along'. Whatever difference the bodywork made, it somehow helped him to *acknowledge* that knowledge, so that by the end of the session it was easier for him to make a cognitive connection between the strange ache between his shoulder blades and the fear of the audience not responding. You could finish a session like this by coming back to the Outcome question one more time: 'And when you've known it all along, **what would you like to have happen now?**' This helps the client to start experimenting with strategies that might be useful to use at the first sign of the symptom recurring, like breathing mindfully into that area.

ASKING WITH SILENCE

In this next example, provided by a colleague who was experimenting with Clean Language, the client has real difficulty finding any positive response to the Clean questions, but the practitioner patiently refuses to give up, not beginning the hands-on bodywork until the client has finally managed to get some positive sense of what he wants.

And what would you like to have happen?
- I just want the pain to go away. (He sits there looking tense and rigid.)

And what kind of pain is it?
- My ankle hurts and my back is always painful. (He sticks out his left foot as he says this, and then brings his right hand to his lower back and lets out a little sigh.)

Where exactly does your back hurt?
- I think it's from all the lifting, moving into my new flat. But it's not that bad. It's my ankle that's really been bothering me.

And where exactly do you feel it?
- Right along here. Maybe I strained it, or maybe it's a joint pain…I don't know, it's just frustrating.

And when you have the pain there, what happens next?
- My whole leg feels weak.

And when the whole leg feels weak, what would you like to have happen?
- I just want the ankle to stop hurting.

At this point I decide that we're going round in circles, and since I can't think of anything else to ask, we just sit together in silence for a moment. Before I can ask another question, he says:

- I need my ankle to loosen up.

At last he has answered the Outcome question in positive language, so I choose the keywords to put into my next Clean question:

*And if it could loosen up, **what would that be like?***
- It would feel more relaxed, less tight probably.

This response clearly shows that the client is beginning to get the idea. Even being able to imagine his ankle loosening up is a step in the right direction, and a move away from the frustration that he is experiencing. So I ask if this would be a good place to begin the treatment. Using a meridian-based approach to assess the imbalance, I find a pattern that reflects not just the joint pain, but also a deep need to recharge his batteries. At the end, the client finds it hard to believe what happened.

How does** the ankle **seem now?
- It's incredible, but it's gone. When you worked on it I could feel the contact from your hand long after you had taken it away. Like it was releasing all by itself. Really weird, but very reassuring. My back is fine now too.

And is there anything else about all that?
- Yes, tiredness, I feel really tired. I spent the whole weekend moving into my new place, in between two really busy weeks at work. Not a great idea, but it felt okay at the time – I was buzzing. Now I just feel exhausted. I could go to sleep right here.

Of course, it's impossible to say how much the Clean questions contributed to this result. Maybe the bodywork could have achieved it on its own. The key point is that through the questions, the client moved from a purely negative view of his symptoms to being able to imagine a positive outcome. Because of that he will now be less likely to think of the treatment as some kind of miracle cure, and more likely to realise that when symptoms do appear, Clean questions are always there as a way of paying more attention to what those symptoms have to say.

THE POWER OF A POSITIVE ANSWER

A client was getting seriously frustrated as she told her shiatsu therapist about a situation at work. Having been a senior manager, she had chosen to take a lower-status job in the same organisation as a break from the burdens of responsibility. Her problem was that her new manager was intimidated by having to manage someone who had only recently been in a very senior executive role, and he had no idea how to handle the situation. As the client talked about her sense of frustration with her manager, her shoulders tightened and her fists clenched.

And where is this frustration?
- Right up to here (she held her hand horizontally across her throat). But I don't let it out, even though every time I see my manager, I want to confront him about it.

Perhaps the Clean questions were making her more aware of just how angry she really was; but she looked as though, if she didn't express it she would have a stroke, and if she did express it she would explode. The practitioner had learned some Clean Language and realised that instead of focusing on the problem, her client needed to start thinking about the solution. So she asked the Outcome question.

And when you don't let it out, even though you want to confront him about it, what would you like to have happen?
- (She looked blank, but only for a moment) Yes, I could go round my manager.

As she said this, she made a gesture with her hand of going around an obstacle. Suddenly, she burst into a broad smile, her cheeks flushed, and she started to laugh. The anger had completely disappeared.

And how would it be to go round your manager?
- I could ask for my old job back.

And what would that be like?
- A relief...that's a surprise!

It turned out that the real issue for the client was her own relationship to her previous senior management job and its high stress levels; her explosive level of frustration was not so much about her current manager's behaviour but her feelings of shame and guilt at having given up her previous job. The Outcome question helped her make a real shift in her attitude towards herself, and the effect of the bodywork was so strong that she had to stand up and sway gently from side to side for about five minutes after it, like a tree bending gently in the wind, experiencing somatically her new sense of her more flexible self.

TO WAKE UP FULLY PRESENT

In this final example, a client who had suffered a near-fatal traffic accident had been having regular bodywork treatments, which she believed had been central to her being able to make an almost complete recovery. Her practitioner was learning Clean Language and decided to try the Outcome question as a way of starting their next session.

And what would you like from this session?
- To feel calm and clear (although there is no real movement or shift in her as she says it).

And what would that be like, to feel calm and clear?
- (Her eyes look up as if in some kind of search) To wake up fully present.

I hadn't heard her say anything quite like that before, and feeling curious I decided to follow it up with one more Clean question.

And is there anything else about wake up fully present?

She hesitated for a few moments, then she took a deep breath in and started to talk in a whole new way about waking up and feeling she was restored to what she remembers as her full former stamina and strength. She got quite excited and talked about her sense of being very close to re-accessing this and how she would then feel somehow younger and strong again. I was thrilled to find her so captivated by the notion of looking at her story in terms of positive outcome rather than ridding herself of negatives.

This is a good example of how, towards the end of a long healing journey, asking the Outcome question can help a client start thinking about future possibilities and feel more able to let go of the trauma of the past. Her deeper breath as she began to do that was literally a kind of 'inspiration', and there is a real sense of shared excitement between client and practitioner here as she begins to explore what 'Wake up fully present' would mean to her.

You've now covered all the basic principles of Clean Language and very nearly finished Part 1. In Part 2 we'll be looking at some of the research into how communication between mind and body actually works, but first, let's set Clean questions free from the very formal boundaries of the client/therapist relationship and see what happens when you have a chance to play a little with what you've learned so far.

$\backsim$ 13 $\backsim$

A CLEAN CONVERSATION

The psychologist Stephen Pinker put it beautifully on the first page of his first best-selling book, *The Language Instinct* (1994). Words, he said, allow us, with 'exquisite precision' to influence what happens in other people's brains: 'By making noises with our mouths, we can reliably cause precise new combinations of ideas to arise in each other's minds. The ability comes so naturally we are apt to forget what a miracle it is' (p.1).

In this first part of the book, you've been learning how to use this miraculous ability in a Clean and mindful way when you talk to your clients. But before we go on to look in more detail at how Clean Language works in clinical practice, I suggest we forget all about the very special rules and dynamics of professional therapeutic relationships and see what happens when we apply some of this 'exquisite precision' to an ordinary conversation between friends. Imagine you've been inspired enough to sign up for a Clean Language course. In class, you've been practising how to use Clean questions to facilitate real positive change with some of your own issues in both mind and body. But now you want to try slipping a few Clean questions into everyday conversations, where the other person doesn't know the rules that you and your fellow students have been following, just to see what happens.

Let's say you're out for a meal with a friend you want to catch up with. You know she's been through some tough times recently; the dream job she got last year descended into nightmare when a new boss took over. You can see the stress in her face, but when you ask her how she's been, she launches with surprising passion into an account of a recent holiday in Spain. As she tells you about an incredibly beautiful beach and the colour of the sea, she really does begin to shape events in your brain. But as well as the images of beach and sea you notice a hint of resentment arising as you think about how long it is since you've had a holiday like that. Not wanting this to show, and finding that the words 'holiday' and 'Spain' have sparked a memory of your own, you nod as enthusiastically as you can and say something about what a great time you had once in Barcelona.

By the tennis match rules of everyday conversation, it's you who have now shaped an event in your friend's brain, since she has to put the image of her beach on pause and mentally click on 'Barcelona' – and any associations that brings up for her – to be able to make sense of what you've just said. But from the sequence of expressions that suddenly appear on her face – a strange medley of polite impatience followed by an attempt to look interested followed in turn by a more fragile look that seems to be saying 'Please listen!' – you can tell that there's something that she really wants to say, so you make a conscious decision to let go of Barcelona and of your resentment too, and suddenly you remember that this may be just the opportunity to try out your Clean questions.

So what did she say? Something about a beach...an amazing beach...no, a beautiful beach, in fact an 'incredibly beautiful beach'. Remember, the first principle in Clean Language is to respect the other person's exact words and to be unusually curious about what those words really mean to them. Treating these words with care, you return them as a question that contains as few of your own ideas as it possibly can. With your friend's fragile look still holding your eye, you simply repeat her keywords and wrap them in a few more, offering her your first Clean question.

And was there anything else about *that incredibly beautiful beach?*

She gives you a slightly surprised look, as if to check that you really are listening now, and starts again on the delicate business of making precise new combinations of ideas arise in your brain.

– Just something about the sea being so clear and blue.

Hardly original, you think, but from the way she says it, she seems to be asking you for help to reconnect with this whole experience. So, curious to know more and setting your judgements aside, you focus again on the words that seemed most important this time – 'clear and blue' – and ask:

And what kind of *clear and blue?*

The question is an invitation to move from mental labels – which are indeed like holiday snapshots – to a deeper, more felt kind of memory. This can take time to upload onto the mental screen, and to be translated into words. Also, these are very visual words and when you say them you notice she closes her eyes as if to see something more clearly inside her head. You also notice her touch her solar plexus with the palm of her right hand.

– It sounds silly, but it just gave me the feeling of being back in my body again.

Hmmm…already this conversation between two friends has got to a delicate point. From a simple dialogue, it's turning into a kind of triangular conversation between you, your friend and something inside her, some more bodily sense of herself. But the way she just told you about being back in her body again – with a slight tilt of the head, eyebrows raised and her voice going up at the end of the sentence – seems like an invitation to try one more.

And what was that like, *being back in your body again?*

As you say this, you notice yourself attending even more closely to her reaction, almost the way someone bowling a ball down a bowling alley follows it with every muscle to see how it hits the pins. There's no knowing, when you bowl a question like this, how it will impact since you're really asking the other person to go well beyond their normal labels for things. That may not be a place they feel ready – or know how – to go to, so you phrase the question carefully, using the same past tense that she used, '**And what was that like…?**' rather than 'And what *is* that like…?', to respect the fact that she is still speaking of it as a memory rather than a present-moment experience. To answer it, she is silent again as her bodymind assembles the different elements of the experience and tries to put them into words. Gazing out of the window, as if she's looking at something a long way off, she takes a deep breath in, flashes a smile and sits up straighter.

– More like me! … Or how I'd like to be, at least.

You notice a mixed message in the way she says this – the first part 'More like me!' looks and sounds very real and direct, as if it's coming from somewhere very alive inside her. But then she looks down, tightens her mouth and speaks more quietly as she says the second part about 'how I'd like to be, at least'. The sentence seems to take her from a stronger connection with herself to a weaker one, almost like a graph that rises steeply, peaks and then slides downwards. This is emphasised by the fact that the first word in the sentence is 'More' and the last one is 'least', which may, of course, be pure coincidence.

Now you're wondering that if you asked another question, would it take her further up or further down? But curious about her sense that she could be more like herself, you push your luck with one more:

And how would that be, to be more like you?
- (Suddenly she looks you straight in the eyes and laughs nervously) I don't know...I'm talking rubbish! What was it like in Barcelona?

Oops...one question too far! You are suddenly back in a normal conversation again, where you agree to listen to your friend's experiences in exchange for her listening to yours. But what really happened there? How was it that with just three questions (yes, just three; go back and count if you don't believe me) you may have helped your friend get to the brink of a real personal insight, and what was it that made her back away again in response to your fourth? Because Clean questions are designed to remove all the usual conversational clutter, and because they focus attention so precisely on what has just been said, response by response, once you start asking them you have to be careful. Like the cartoon character suspended in that mid-air moment of realising there's nothing underneath but empty space, in any conversation (everyday ones as well as therapeutic ones), it's quite common to find you've talked the other person over the edge of whatever solid ground they normally inhabit.

Clean Language is particularly good at doing this; it's what it's designed for, which is why it's important to have some kind of safety net in place when you start asking Clean questions, something that gives your friend or client the choice of whether to go on, stay where they are, or go back. Your friend made her own decision to drop the subject and return to normal conversation. Between a client and a practitioner, that sort of behaviour can easily be labelled as resistant or a sign of inner conflict, but in any conversation it is also possible that it's simply not the time or place or you are not the person they want to have it with. Clean Language, well used, leaves that to the client, and reminds the practitioner again and again to respect that choice. After all, in the conversation you just had, it's possible that simply going over that edge and being able to get back again was much more help to her than you might realise.

Just then the food arrives: a warm aubergine salad sprinkled with feta cheese and finely chopped mint for your friend, while you have slow-braised squid with fennel and coriander served with oven-crisped slices of baguette brushed with a little olive oil. As you eat with your friend, by mutual consent absorbing yourselves in the tastes and textures, the succulent softness of the squid or the crusty crunch of the bread, you are both also quietly digesting what's been said so far.

Did I succeed in shaping some events in your brain just then? Did you notice a mental shift as your mind suddenly needed to process words about taste and smell and texture, using different parts of your brain from the very language-focused words that came before? If you want you can read them again, imagining yourself smelling and tasting those flavours, and notice the effect it has somatically.

After a few minutes' eating silently together, your friend fixes you with a quizzical look and asks, 'What were all those questions you were asking me, anyway?' Oh dear, and you thought you'd slipped your Clean questions in so conversationally that she hadn't even noticed them. People usually do notice when you use more than one or two Clean questions in a row, if only because it creates a completely different sense of being listened to than normal conversation. So as you tell her about the course you're doing and try to explain what Clean Language is, she suddenly interrupts.

- Go on then, ask me another one.

About what?
- About what I was talking about before.

You remember from the course how useful it can be to summarise what someone has already said, and you try to remember all her keywords.

There was an incredibly beautiful beach where the sea was so clear and blue, and that gave you the feeling of being back in your body, and when you're back in your body, you're more...euh...

She looks at you, nodding, as if giving permission for you to ask the question she shied away from before. This time, you ask it a little differently.

*More like you. **And when** you're more like you, **that's like what?***

You know all about how powerful metaphors can be as a way of helping people connect with their inner landscape of feeling and meaning, so the question you've asked is a direct invitation to find one. She rests her elbows on the table and folds her arms in front of her, looking straight down at the tablecloth. To your surprise, her jaw tightens and when she looks up again, her smile has gone.

- I don't know. I've got this new boss and she's reorganising everything and I'm getting more and more anxious. Is she going to get rid of me, or what? I'm having nightmares about it, and these panicky reactions, like even if I see an email from her in my inbox...

Wait a minute...this isn't what she was supposed to say. Instead of coming up with a metaphor for this positive sense of being more like herself, your question seems to have sent her in the opposite direction, to what it's like being anxious and panicky. As a good friend you would normally do your best to listen. But this time you're surprised to find you're holding up your hand to interrupt her. Even though you didn't get the metaphor you were hoping for, you know what to ask next. Just follow the basic rule, take what she just said, and ask another question. You decide to experiment with one you haven't used very much yet.

And what happens just before *that panicky reaction when you see an email from her in your inbox?*

She looks at you for a moment, trying to make sense of the question.

− I tighten up.

And where do you tighten up?

She gestures to her solar plexus, the same place she touched when she first mentioned feeling 'more like me'.

And then what happens?

You see her face go blank, then pink, and she seems to have stopped breathing. It's as if her body has heard your question but her head doesn't know how to answer.

− I don't know. It just goes all tight and I get really angry...I just feel completely stuck!

As she says this she sounds on the brink of tears. You feel your heart going out to her and want to help, and at the same time you're beginning to panic a bit yourself. Then something one of your teachers said about what to do when your client seems stuck comes back to you: it's probably you that's stuck, not your client. You notice that you've stopped breathing too. You're wondering if you should just tell her to take a few deep breaths, forget about Clean Language and get back to the meal, when another question pops into your head:

And what needs to happen when it goes all tight and you get really angry?

What comes out next really is a surprise. Through gritted teeth, she emits a livid growl:

− I need to kill my fucking boss!

You look at each other, both slightly shocked. For a moment, she looks as though she really means it. In all the years you've known her, you've never experienced her murderous side before. But even if you're worried that your Clean questions have set off some kind of chain reaction inside her, what else can you do but ask another question?

And when *you kill your fucking boss,* **then what happens?**

She stares over your shoulder as if watching a movie she's never seen before, then surprises you with her answer:

- She'd have more respect for me.

And when *she has more respect for you,* **then what happens?**

She puts her hand back on her solar plexus, the same place it went to right at the beginning when she was talking about how the clear, blue sea gave her the feeling of being back in her body again.

- I have a bit more respect for *her*, I suppose. Less fear. I can see where she's coming from.

You're beginning to realise that in the world of Clean Language, anything can happen. If your friend or client has to murder someone, that's okay. At least it's a Clean kill, which means that it may only take another question or two to bring them back to life. Clean logic emerges in its own way. All you have to do is to stay out of its way.

And when *you can see where she's coming from,* **then what happens?**
- I can just get on with my job, but like a grown-up.

And is there anything else about *like a grown-up?*

She is silent for a while as she processes your invitation to explore this adult sense of self. As usual, her response comes first through the body – she shifts in her chair, sitting up a little straighter, aligning her spine and lifting her chin.

- Yes, then I'm more like me again, just like I said before.

Her hand already told you that three questions ago when it went back to her solar plexus where this 'More like me' seems to have its somatic location. But now she has made a conscious connection with what she said all the way back at the beginning of the conversation.

And when *you're more like you,* ***then what happens?***
- It's good.

And where is *good?*
- Here.

She touches her solar plexus again and takes a deep breath in, closing her eyes and disappearing one more time into her internal landscape.

And is there anything else about *a deep breath there?*

She nods, then smiles, as if a rather long and complicated joke has finally reached its punch-line.

- Clear blue sea!

She opens her eyes. You look at each other. She looks very different: the muscles of her eyes and jaw are at ease, not on alert; her face has a genuinely peaceful look; and for the moment at least, in some indefinable way, she really does seem to have that 'more like me' quality about her.

Of course, the proof of the pudding will only emerge when she's back at work, or maybe when she sees another email from her boss in her inbox. Clean Language is not about solving people's problems for them: it's about helping them explore and map as accurately as possible, somatically as well as psychologically, the internal landscape of any particular issue. It's also about trusting that they will be able to make connections there between things that haven't been connected before.

Just as you would with a client at the end of a bodywork session, it may help to spend a little time going over what happened, and helping her to notice what her body has been telling her – the way her hand moved to her solar plexus, and how that very important centre of body-energy seems to be a real resource, connecting her to the felt sense of what the image of the 'clear, blue sea' is really all about. You may also ask what she could do next time she stops breathing when she sees an email from her boss in her inbox. For example, to pause, bring her hand to her solar plexus, remind herself that she's a grown-up, visualise that clear blue sea and just stay mindfully present with her sensations until her normal breathing starts again. New connections have been made, and the practical difference is that when she feels that panic again, she now has a panic button. There may be more she needs to do, but a genuinely useful piece of work has been done, and you and your Clean questions helped her do it.

14

A CLEAN CONVERSATION:
WHAT DID YOU LEARN?

So you survived and your friend survived and hopefully her boss did too. Your curiosity about trying out a few Clean questions may have got you into deeper water than you were expecting, but you held on to the lifeline which is always there in Clean – taking whatever the other person has just said and putting it into another Clean question – and helped her to cross a river that she'd never crossed before. Okay, enough metaphors. What did you learn from all that? Here are nine key points to take with you as you practise your Clean questions with other people and through the rest of this book:

1. TELL PEOPLE WHAT YOU'RE DOING

When you start learning how to use Clean Language, it's like learning any other language – there's a lot to think about and you know you'll be making mistakes as part of the process. If you want to practise your Greek or your English or your Mandarin with a native speaker, you'd usually explain first that you're a beginner and ask them for their help. In the same way, if you explain to your clients that you're learning a new way of asking questions and ask if they'd be willing to try it, you're doing at least three important things to make it easier for you and more effective for them. First, you're taking some of the pressure off. If they look blank, or you forget what to ask, or you start to feel out of your depth, you can just thank them for being willing to experiment, make a mental note of what you learned, and move on.

Second, no matter how informally you ask your Clean questions, people will almost always realise that you're using a very different kind of language, simply because to answer your questions they have to go to parts of their brain they don't usually go to. If you get their permission first, then you engage their interest and cooperation rather than their suspicion.

Third, if they're expecting some kind of body or energy work from you, you're changing the contract between you if you start asking more than one or two Clean questions in a row. One practitioner who studied with me tried her Clean questions on a client who was a psychotherapist. By the time she got to the **'What would you like to have happen?'** question, he was looking distinctly uncomfortable. The simple bodywork that he valued so much seemed to him to have been replaced by an attempt at some kind of talking therapy and he told the practitioner that this wasn't part of the contract he'd agreed to. When she explained that the questions were to help them 'co-create an appropriate energetic field' for the bodywork, it made sense to him and he agreed to try this new way of listening to himself. They soon discovered a key gesture that provided a link between the story he was telling and the way his body was being affected by it, and he realised how useful Clean questions could be. But he was right to say that the contract had been changed, and by asking for permission first, you make that plain.

2. WHATEVER HAPPENS, ACCEPT IT

In answer to your second Clean question, your friend said, 'It sounds silly, but it just gave me the feeling of being back in my body again.' In a normal conversation, we pretend to know what people mean when they say things like this – it keeps things moving along at a safe and superficial level. But one thing that Clean Language teaches you is that you actually have no idea what 'back in my body again' really means to the person saying it – and most probably neither do they until you ask them. It may sound like a good sort of place to be, and it certainly raises the question of where she was before she was back in her body, but asking Clean questions is a dynamic process, not an intellectual interrogation. It depends more than anything else on the sense of trust she has in where the questions are taking her, a trust that can easily be weakened if the person asking them is treating it as just a game or an exercise.

Whatever your client says in answer to a Clean question, it's not your job to judge whether it makes sense, or how useful or even how ethical that answer may be. In Clean Language, the customer is always right. Even if it sounds shocking, remember they are speaking from their own very subjective internal virtual reality, where anything can happen. They will almost certainly be as surprised as you to hear what they have just said, and that is the whole point. You are simply there to facilitate and guide that process of 'self-listening'. If you do ignore or reject something they say, and deliberately decide not to include it in your next question, then at some level your client will notice that and their trust in your ability to really listen to them deeply and with full acceptance may wobble.

3. COMPLETING THE CIRCLE

When blood can't flow properly to some part of the body, bodywork can help to restore the circulation. In the same way, Clean Language helps the client to clear any blocks that are in the way of the free flow of energy, thought and emotion associated with some particular issue. In your friend's case this was building up into a stagnated lump of emotion that was only able to express itself in her nightmares. Thanks to your questions, it suddenly erupted into the conversation, perhaps because at some deep level she knew that Clean questions made that safe. Once it was released, energy was able to flow again around that particular circuit of her bodymind but in a new way. When your client hits a brick wall, instead of thinking that the wall is impenetrable, it can be much more helpful to think of it simply as a part of a circuit that needs to flow more freely. And if, with Clean Language, the client is able to find a way through, over, around or under that wall, the next time her energy flows around that circuit, it will know there is now a way through a part that was completely blocked before.

4. EXPECT THE UNEXPECTED

There's no point trying to second guess your client, or to think you've been there before; they will always come up with something weirder than you can. The more you try to shepherd them along a certain path, the less they will have the freedom to explore the fascinating details of their internal landscape which, remember, you are only ever experiencing at second hand. Only they can see it, sense it, hear and feel it.

5. BE AN ADVOCATE FOR THE BODYMIND

Your client may need your help believing in the responses they find themselves giving to your questions. Their answers may sound strange, clichéd, childish, incoherent or even threatening to their everyday sense of self. Encourage them not to censor them and remember that the verbal mind will often say, 'I don't know,' before the answer has had time to emerge. Be a patient listener, and they will learn from you.

6. THE BODY NEVER LIES

Use Clean questions like, '**What just happened?**' to bring your client's attention to their unconscious gestures, changes in breathing and posture and other subtle hints their bodymind is trying to give them. Gently make your clients aware of the fact that, while they may often find it hard to put something into words, their gestures are almost always 100 per cent accurate as a description of what is really going on at the somatic and energetic level.

7. WHEN IN DOUBT, BAIL OUT

Above all, remember how quickly Clean questions can bring up surprising metaphors or unfamiliar somatic sensations, and respect your client's sense of safety. When the bodymind tries to drag your client into some unresolved trauma, their immediate reaction is often to pull away from it, to reject, deny or repress it in some way. They will need a lot of faith in your patience and skill to feel safe enough to accept that there's something important there and that they can deal with it. One way to build that trust is to remind them that they can stop the process at any time. If they start to look uncomfortable, ask them if that would be a good place to press the pause button and take a breath. Often just knowing that you are aware that they are finding something challenging will give your client more confidence to carry on. If it seems like they need to recover their equilibrium, you can always come back to the Outcome question, '**And with all of that, what would you like to have happen?**' to help them reconnect with the positive aspects of the issue and recover a sense of agency.

8. SO WHAT ABOUT THE BODYWORK...?

So if a few Clean questions can achieve so much without any actual bodywork, why put Clean Language together with bodywork therapy? Why not just leave them as separate disciplines? Well, wait a minute; who says there was no bodywork? As soon as we begin to speak about anything that really matters to us, our eyes, face, lips, tongue, vocal cords, hands, posture and breathing all become involved. The client's body is working long before we start using any formal bodywork techniques. In fact, the first use of touch often comes from the client – in this case when your friend unconsciously touched her solar plexus with the palm of her hand as she thought about being back in her body again. Working in a Clean way with our clients includes noticing and accepting all the information they offer us, and helping them realise how much their own body is already communicating the subtleties of habitual thoughts and spontaneous insights. Then any bodywork techniques you introduce already have a firm foundation in the client's reality.

9. AND WHAT ABOUT THE FOOD...?

What was so important about getting you to notice that shift from reading about words to reading about tastes and smells and textures? To answer this, think for a moment about the difference between how you might feel when you're talking about a problem that's really worrying you, and how you'd feel enjoying the flow of conversation as you share a meal with friends. When we're concerned and anxious, the body keeps us alert, tense and ready for action. When we feel comfortable, we are able to nourish ourselves both through relationships and through what the body can absorb, whether through food or through touch. In Clean Language, your presence and intentions help to create that nourishing atmosphere, but when you make the body the primary focus of the work, it is like bringing food to the table. Conversation may continue to flow, but there is something else going on, something beyond the words, which allows the bodymind to settle comfortably into the embrace of its own awareness. When you mix Clean Language with bodywork therapy, sometimes the Clean questions can be a tempting starter, sometimes a good dessert; sometimes they can accompany it like wine with a meal, but the bodywork is usually the main course.

The point of building this sense of safety and connectedness is not just to give your clients a holiday from their troubles. The point is to give them the support that they need to be able to approach those troubles with the acceptance, confidence and curiosity that will help them take the next step in their process of self-healing. As we saw in that conversation with your friend, often we need to go back and forth between the challenging and the convivial, between the difficult and the comforting, several times in one session.

In facilitating this movement back and forth between the defended and the vulnerable we are reflecting what the body does naturally in releasing itself from trauma; and what we can offer our clients through touch, contact and awareness of movement is as vital as anything we can do with Clean Language. Our challenge is to get the balance right between language and touch, so that clients not only discover how their own words can lead them into the surprising and unfamiliar world of somatic intelligence; they can also translate these mysterious metaphorical messages and sensations into words that make sense to the everyday mind – that part of us that is so essential in planning, organising and implementing the strategies that we need to achieve our outcomes, whatever those outcomes may be.

PART 2
THE THEORY

~ 15 ~

THE SCIENCE BEHIND
CLEAN LANGUAGE

When we use Clean Language in mind/body therapy, what is really happening? How is it that simply by holding symptoms in awareness and using Clean questions to focus and channel attention, long-held patterns can begin to change, not only in the mind but in the body too? How can language have such a direct effect on our physiology and energy systems? And can neuroscience, or the new science of embodied cognition, or any other kind of science for that matter, offer us objective explanations for a process that seems to the logical mind to be so utterly subjective and impossible to measure or test? If, as Iain McGilchrist has said, 'Science is neither more nor less than patient and detailed attention to the world' (2010, p.7), then the best way I can answer this is to invite you on a brief journey through the work of three pioneers of the science of mind/body communication. All of them highly respected in their own fields, each has had the courage to link different academic disciplines together, and even to think *between* disciplines, as we must if we want to explore how living systems really work.

So here in Part 2 we look at some of the theory behind what happens when we use Clean Language to help our clients connect mind, brain and body. If you are more interested in the practical applications of Clean Language, then feel free to skip this section, or to come back to it later when your curiosity gets the better of you. Also I should emphasise that this is in no way intended as any kind of unified theory of psycho-physiological intelligence. The scientific way of exploring the world is beginning to build shared meanings with what Dan Siegel, clinical professor of psychiatry at the UCLA School of Medicine, calls the 'wisdom traditions' that many forms of bodywork are rooted in. But you would have to read a lot more than I can offer here to get a comprehensive overview of that literature – and there would be no better place to start than with the work of Dan Siegel himself, author of the brilliantly interdisciplinary *Mindsight* (2010). But the work of each of these three pioneers is a major tributary to what has become a fast-flowing river: the study of how, and how much, we influence each other somatically as well as cognitively when we communicate. When we use Clean Language to communicate with the body, whether we know it or not, we are stepping into this new field of 'interpersonal neurobiology'. So this section is meant simply as a brief introduction to one practical process and two current theories that offer some insight into what might be happening when we try to use language to go beyond words.

⮑ 16 ⮐

FOCUSING THE MIND
ON THE BODY

As a boy in 1938, Eugene Gendlin began a desperate journey with his Jewish family to escape from Nazi-occupied Vienna. That same year another more famous fugitive, Sigmund Freud, then 82, only managed to escape because of his international fame and diplomatic connections. Eleven-year-old Eugene's father, with no such connections, had to rely on a different but equally valuable kind of resource: his ability to listen to what his body was telling him. At one point in their long and complex route via Germany to Holland, his father had to negotiate with a man who was offering them an apartment to hide in. Young Eugene sat outside the room while they talked. Finally his father came out, looking pale. All he said was, 'Let's go'. In the street outside, his father explained that he didn't trust the man. When Eugene asked him why, his father simply repeated something he had often said before, 'I follow my feeling,' and this time his feeling said 'No'. The boy was puzzled that his father had abandoned what seemed like their only hope of safety for nothing more than a feeling. He wondered what kind of feelings could hold such information and how you got to have them (Korbei 2007).

Forty years later, Gendlin, by then a psychologist at the University of Chicago and a student and then colleague of Carl Rogers, the founder of person-centred therapy, had found his answer. In his best-selling book *Focusing*, first published in 1978, he gave a vivid example of how he used this subtle, non-verbal, embodied way of knowing to help a young woman caught in a negative spiral of suicidal thoughts (pp.11–16).

FINDING THE FELT SENSE

When she phoned him one day desperate for help, she had paced the streets all morning, afraid that she was pregnant from yet another casual encounter with a man she had no feelings for. Having worked with her before, Gendlin gently but firmly tried to talk her down, literally deeper down inside herself to find the 'felt sense' of all this. But it didn't work. Realising that her head was so full it was stopping her from connecting with her body, he asked her instead just to clear enough space in her mind to be able to look at what was going on in there, to find the problems and look at them one by one. The phone went quiet, then she said that what hurt most was not her fear of being pregnant but something from many years before – losing the only man she'd ever really loved. This triggered another flow of tearful self-destructive thoughts.

Interrupting, Gendlin invited her again to go deeper down inside to 'the unclear body sense of it all'. Again there was silence. Then a word popped into her head, 'Anger'. It was a surprise to her. This anger was not a familiar feeling, so she went back and forth between the word and what she sensed in her body to check that it was right. It was. She started to ask herself why she should be angry, but he encouraged her instead to ask the felt sense directly what this anger was about. Silence again. Then at last, he heard her sigh – something had shifted. She was angry with herself, she said, for sleeping with a man who only wanted her for sex.

As she said this, she noticed a change in what she felt inside and looked for a word for this new feeling: 'Weary!' Gendlin could hear the relief in her voice as she realised this was her most deeply felt body sense, and that it was an expression of her deepest fear – that she would spend the rest of her life in lifeless relationships. In her mind's eye, she said, she could see, 'All those men lined up ahead of me, all those blank faces, rows and rows of them from here to the end of my life.'

To Gendlin's surprise, she was so relieved at this discovery that she felt their session was done. Logically, he thought, nothing had really changed in her situation, so what gave her the feeling that something had indeed changed at some deeper level? And what gave Gendlin the confidence that the most effective way to help a potentially suicidal woman, who could easily have hung up on him at any moment, was to ask her to start rummaging around inside herself for unclear felt sensations?

LOST FOR WORDS

The answer is the many years of research that he and his colleagues had already done, listening to recordings of thousands of hours of psychotherapy sessions in an attempt to find out why therapy only seemed to work for some clients, while others were left with no real change in their feelings or their lives. This very obvious question was not one that most psychotherapists at that time were keen to ask. The prevailing, almost religiously held belief, according to Gendlin, was that therapy was an art, not a science, not just for the therapist but for the client too. Failure to benefit from therapy (which research showed was the experience of the majority of clients) was simply a sign that the client had no aptitude for it. But as Gendlin and his colleagues listened to recordings of thousands of therapy sessions, they began to notice a startling pattern, one so clear that it enabled them to predict from just one or two sessions whether or not the therapy would work. The clients who did benefit from therapy would invariably at some point in a session find themselves lost for words. As Ann Weiser Cornell, an early student and later colleague of Gendlin's puts it, they would, 'Slow down their talk, become less articulate and begin groping for words to describe something that they were feeling at the moment' (Cornell 1996, p.5).

Whatever they were feeling, the fact that it was so difficult to put this bodily awareness into words intrigued Gendlin, and for a very good reason. When he first joined Carl Rogers as a psychology student he already had a PhD in philosophy, and the philosophical question that most fascinated him was how the constructs, symbols and sensations which make up our inner reality interact with and shape our experience of the apparently objective world beyond our skin. If all our sensory information comes to us through our bodily senses, how do we translate that into words?

Gendlin brought a radical mix of interdisciplinary curiosity and intellectual courage to his research, and his philosopher's intuition suggested to him that underneath the physical symptoms and specific emotions which we usually have words for (and may be encouraged by our therapist to 'get in touch with'), there had to be a deeper, non-verbal somatic way of understanding our lived experience. Maybe that's what these clients were connecting with as they groped for words. Realising that neither everyday language nor the language of therapy had words to describe it, he had to invent his own. His first attempts did not trip off the tongue. 'Direct referant' and 'preconceptual feeling' were early terms he used to describe this embodied way of knowing.[1] Eventually he came up with a term which has become so much a part of everyday language that few who use it realise that it refers to something much more subtle than just a physical sensation or a particular emotion. 'Felt sense' was the term, and the process of discovering and communicating with this felt sense is now well known to many mind/body therapists as 'Focusing'.

---

1   Gendlin, E.T. and Cornell, A.W. *Conversations at the Edge*. Online phone seminar, 19 February 2015.

PAYING ATTENTION TO WHAT IS NOT YET CLEAR

He described the felt sense as something different from a symptom or an emotion, something that would only emerge if you took the time and paid enough attention in the right kind of way. Though some people do this intuitively, he did not pretend that it was easy to learn. The point of Focusing was to show that it *could* be learned, and to help people do that he devised a six-step process for connecting with it and communicating with it. After four decades of development, he and other Focusing teachers now describe this tuning-in to the felt sense as a more fluid process in which all the steps may be happening at the same time to some degree. But as Focusing evolves, what remains at the core of the process is the 'zigzag': this going back and forth between the 'felt sense' and the words, images or movements that emerge to describe it; the waiting for a resonance between them; and the internal response, the 'felt shift', which is the body's way of saying that something has changed inside.

In the foreword to *Focusing* (Gendlin 1978, p.xi), Marilyn Ferguson, who was herself a best-selling writer on the mind and the brain, wondered if the 'felt shift' might have to do with the fact that the two sides of the brain communicate with the body in different ways. In the 40 years since she wrote that, neuroscientists largely ignored the question – until recently. In Chapter 18 we'll look at that more recent research in detail. What's important now is that the spirit of Clean Language – the respect for the client's precise words – takes us right back to Gendlin's original research and his fine-tuned ear for the ways that language can either help or hinder this delicate and intimate process of connecting with one's own inner felt sense. Well before Clean Language came along, he had already made a radical commitment to avoid interpreting or paraphrasing the client's words as most therapists did (and do), and to respect those words as exactly as possible as the essential currency of therapeutic dialogue.

So when we ask Clean questions, the same applies, and especially in those moments when language itself seems to slip away and clients begin to speak more slowly, or close their eyes, or just sound, uh…you know…mmm…less articulate. This loss of articulacy is a sure sign that the speech centre in the left side of the brain has gone into search mode; that it's realised it doesn't have the labels to provide any kind of ready-made description for the new information that's coming from the whole of the rest of the body and brain. Most people experience this as a moment when the mind goes blank – that state of embarrassed empty-mindedness that Zen koans are supposed to induce. Many clients will find it enjoyable, or even entrancing (literally) to find themselves temporarily lost for words but completely absorbed in that tip-of-the-tongue sense (in the poet Philip Larkin's beautiful phrase), of 'something almost being said' (Larkin 2003, p.124). For others, the blankness can at first be irritating, when the well-trod mental corridors they are used to hurrying along suddenly disappear and they're still in a hurry but there's nowhere to go. For others again, this blankness can seem like a no-man's land which they will need your help to cross. Especially if trauma is involved, it can be a genuinely frightening place, and they will have to learn a few skills before they can even approach it. As Ann Weiser Cornell points out in *Focusing in Clinical Practice* (2013), it is a tribute to Gendlin's sensitivity to language that Focusing has inspired 'much of the somatically oriented mindfulness-based work being done today,' including leading approaches like Peter Levine's Somatic Experiencing and Pat Ogden's Sensorimotor Therapy. This brings us to the work of our second mind/body pioneer, a psychiatrist with unusual insight into the role that the nervous system plays in the way we build relationships, including the ones we build with our clients to help them feel safe enough to stay with what is not yet clear.

～ 17 ～

FROM BODY TO BRAIN

If this ability to go back and forth between words and felt sensations is essential to both Focusing and Clean Language, what do we know about how body and brain between them produce – or sometimes fail to produce – the right words to describe what is going on inside us? How exactly does information flow between our conscious mind and our physical body so that words can be translated into feelings and feelings into words…and which comes first, the feelings or the words?

To think that the answer to this question is a simple linear one – that a feeling somewhere inside us has a corresponding word in the brain to describe it – is to miss an essential part of what the question is all about. Spoken language is not just a collection of symbols, a mental semaphore by which meaning is flashed from mind to mind. Humans may be the only creatures to have developed verbal language, but other mammals have highly developed ways of communicating with each other, and the anatomy and neurology we use to speak and listen to language is a product of our evolution as a species. Just as the brain itself, from the cortex on top to the brainstem at the base, reflects the whole history of evolution, so also our ability to speak and understand verbal language depends on a number of systems, some ancient that we share with other species and some which only humans have.

A PLACE OF SAFETY

So where is the best place to start looking for these links between our animal ability to sense things in the raw and our human capacity to express them in words and metaphor? It may be surprising, but according to Dr Stephen Porges, that place has to be where any effective therapy starts, the sense of feeling safe – how safe your client feels in their own body, how safe they feel with you, and how safe you feel with them. Thanks to Porges' *Polyvagal Theory* (2011), we now have a better understanding of how the brain, via a complex set of nerves known as the vagus, may both facilitate and sabotage our efforts as mind/body therapists.

In many kinds of body-energy work, clients often experience a deep sense of being fully present in the body and unusually relaxed in the mind. But at some point in a session, we may also bring them into contact with parts of themselves they have been avoiding for a long time. In a moment, the client's nervous system shifts into alarm mode or freeze mode; they may jerk their hand away from your touch, tense up physically or shut down emotionally. Porges' ground-breaking research on the multiple roles of the vagus nerve suggests how intimately connected these apparently opposite parts of the nervous system might be.

Porges suggests that there are actually three different parts of the vagus that date from different periods of our evolution as a species. The first part does most of the work in conveying internal visceral sensations from body to brain; through it the brain monitors what is going on inside the body and it's probably via this part that the basic ingredients of a 'felt sense' first come into consciousness. The second part of the vagus nerve goes in the opposite direction, from the brain to our internal organs, slowing us down when we need to rest, relax, digest and restore ourselves when weary or worn out. But this slowing-down has another function too, for use only in emergencies: the evolutionarily ancient response to life-threatening danger of 'playing dead'. As we shall see, this works well if you're a reptile, but humans who experience this 'freeze-or-faint' response in traumatic situations, and are unable to release it, can suffer serious consequences – depression, dissociation and fatigue, as well as physical symptoms like irritable bowel syndrome and fibromyalgia. When this primitive response takes over, it is even possible, through cardiac arrest, literally to die of fright. The third and most evolved part of the vagus is our first line of defence against the freeze/faint response. It's an important pathway for signals from the brain that regulate the heart and lungs to restore calm when we start to feel anxiety, unease, aggression or panic in response to internal thoughts or external events. It is also, Porges suggests, a key part of the neural network through which we convey the signals of safety that allow us to connect and bond with our fellow human beings.

THE WANDERING NERVE

The vagus nerve is best known as the largest nerve in the autonomic nervous system – the part of the nervous system that works mainly below the level of conscious control to regulate internal body functions. The vagus plays a major role in letting the brain know how the body is feeling. It takes its name from the Latin word for 'wandering' – the same root is there in 'vagabond' and 'vague'. This may be more than an etymological detail, since Gendlin often speaks of the 'felt sense' as being 'vague' (1978, p.55). To do its job of linking all the body's major organs to the brain it has to snake its way upwards from belly to brainstem, connecting with intestines, cervix, uterus (or testicles and prostate), kidneys, liver, stomach, spleen, pancreas, heart and lungs on the way. The vagus and its branches account for about 80 per cent of the parasympathetic nervous system, and 80 per cent of the information that travels through this nerve goes upwards to the brain. This makes it by far the most important single channel by which sensations that seem to come, say, from the guts or the heart, can reach the brain. When someone asks you that all-important Clean question, '**And where is…?**' about any internal physical or emotional experience, the answer that eventually pops into your head will almost certainly have come via the vagus nerve.

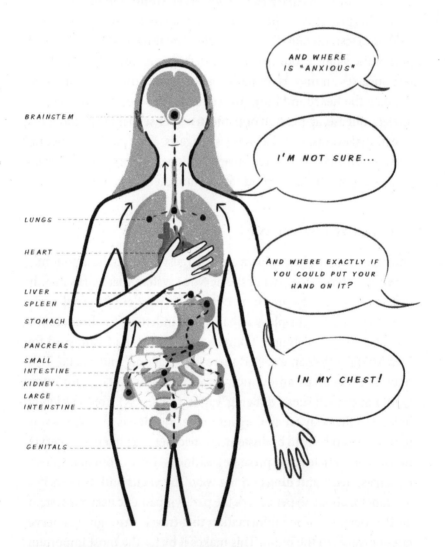

The polyvagal theory: 1 From body to brain

CHIEF NOURISHER

The vagus is not one nerve but a set of nerves originating in different areas of the brainstem with different functions, which is why Porges uses the word 'polyvagal' to describe it. Besides the 80 per cent of the vagus which is 'afferent', bringing somatic information to the brain, it has two 'efferent' branches which send motor signals to the body from the brain. The older one, in evolutionary terms, we share not only with other mammals but also with reptiles and most vertebrates. It does what the vagus is best known for: activating the parasympathetic nervous system, that part of the autonomic nervous system that helps us to rest, digest, recover, heal and grow. Shakespeare's phrase 'Chief nourisher in life's feast' (*Macbeth*, Act 2, Scene 2) is a good description for this part of the vagus, since it connects mainly with the organs below the diaphragm (with some connections to the heart as well), and plays a key role in allowing us to slow down enough for healthy digestion to take place, as blood flow is diverted from the limbs to the gut. The phrase 'a hearty meal' gives a sense of the relaxed satisfaction that we feel when this older part of the vagus is activated, enabling us to feel safely comfortable with ourselves and with our companions at the table.

In contrast, the more recently evolved part of the vagus operates above the diaphragm and connects with the muscles of the heart, throat, larynx, jaw, tongue, ear and face – the muscles which are so important in listening and communication. This more-evolved branch accounts for only 3 per cent of the fibres of the vagus, and these fibres are covered with an insulating layer of myelin, allowing nerve signals to travel much faster than in the older reptilian part of the vagus, which is unmyelinated. This more modern, rapid-reaction part of the vagus regulates the heart and lungs in response to sudden external events and provides an essential link between the heart, the voice, the face and the brain that allows us to exchange social signals of safety.

ENGAGE AND ARTICULATE

Porges calls this part of the vagus, along with the circuits in the brainstem that control it, the 'Social Engagement System' (2011, p.125) since it affects the way we listen, through its connection with the bones and muscles of the inner ear, and also how we speak, through the muscles of the larynx and pharynx. In addition, it connects via the brainstem with the striated (voluntary) muscles of the face and head. Without this more recently evolved part of our neuro-anatomy, the natural mammalian processes of nourishment, communication and attachment between mothers and caregivers on the one hand, and newborns and infants on the other, would be impossible. The same system is important in determining how effective our therapeutic language can be, because it controls our human ability to connect with other people through words, voice tone and facial expression (see figure on page 153).

When all three parts of the polyvagal system are working well together, we feel somatically at ease via the sensory connections from our internal organs to the brain, and the function of these organs is well regulated by the brain via the older motor vagus. Meanwhile the more evolved mammalian/human version gives us the subtle range of skills we need to carry on a conversation. The writer Virginia Woolf seems to have understood all this intuitively in a famous passage from *A Room of One's Own*. She describes how our ability to relax somatically and our ability to relax socially go hand in hand and regulate each other: 'The human frame being what it is, heart, body, and brain all mixed together, and not contained in separate compartments...a good dinner is of importance to good talk. One cannot think well, love well, sleep well, if one has not dined well' (Woolf 1929/1998, p.23).

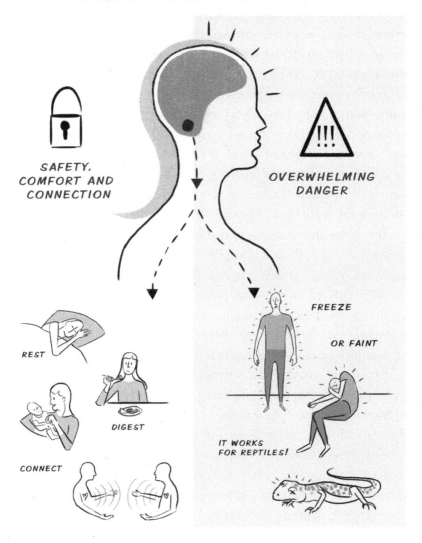

THE SECOND PART OF THE VAGUS NERVE:
SLOWING DOWN OR PLAYING DEAD?

SAFETY, COMFORT AND CONNECTION

OVERWHELMING DANGER

REST

DIGEST

CONNECT

FREEZE

OR FAINT

IT WORKS FOR REPTILES!

The polyvagal theory: 2 From brain to body

HUNKERING DOWN

But there will also be times – say at a dinner where you don't know everyone and maybe find yourself starting to argue with someone whose outspoken views have been irritating you all evening – when the opposite process begins to happen. Maybe your jaw tightens a little, or you find yourself chewing harder on your food. Although consciously you may still be trying to be polite, unconsciously the space between your eyebrows starts to tighten and you begin to look at your antagonist across the table more as a target than a companion. As this fight-or-flight response begins to take over, of course, the person at whom you're directing it is probably going through the same kind of physiological hunkering-down.

This is the atavistic energy that we summon up every time the bodymind begins to shift into a fight-or-flight response. Nowadays, even though the battlefield is usually a metaphorical one, the raw power of this reaction (which comes not via the vagus but via the spinal nerves of the sympathetic nervous system) can quickly turn a stranger into an enemy, sending the mind into a frantic search for memories and associations that will confirm this. And there are only two ways out. One is to attempt to re-engage the more evolved part of the polyvagal system, using words and facial expressions of friendliness and conciliation. Almost certainly, other people at the table will start trying to do this, maybe through humour, or by changing the subject. This appeals to the brain's frontal cortex to get back to doing what it normally does, which is the unconscious inhibition of the fight-or-flight response. This is why paramedics are trained to make eye contact and ask simple direct questions to traumatised patients. That way they calm the patient by making them re-engage through ear, voice and face-to-face contact with their more highly evolved mental functions and restore a coherent relationship between heart and brain.

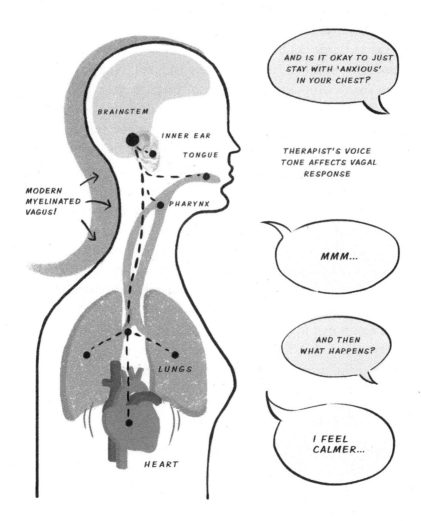

The polyvagal theory: 3 The Social Engagement System – calming and connecting

The second way out of a situation which the brain perceives as a threat brings us to the vagus nerve's other, more sinister role, which derives from the older reptilian part and is so powerful that it can override not only our desire to be social and convivial, but also the sympathetic nervous system's adrenal surge to fight/flight. This freeze/faint response (see figure on page 151) evolved to help smaller creatures avoid the jaws of larger ones, not by turning on their opponent in a fight they couldn't win or by running from a predator who might be faster than them, but by simply playing dead, and so, perhaps, disappearing from the predator's movement-oriented field of vision. This response first evolved in reptiles, whose brains need far less oxygen than mammals' brains do, and who can afford to be immobilised for some time without harm. The freeze/faint reaction is a lot less use to humans, and indeed is potentially lethal if the massive slowing of the heart rate and suspension of breathing that are essential to this immobilisation response mean that oxygen is denied to the brain for too long. It remains wired in to our nervous system as a last-ditch reaction to situations that, for any reason real or imagined, threaten to be overwhelming and from which there's no escape.

THE HIERARCHY OF RESPONSE

Porges suggests that rather than thinking as we usually do of the sympathetic and parasympathetic systems as being in a state of balance or 'paired antagonism', we should instead think of a hierarchical response to perceived threats. First we use the Social Engagement System, the most highly evolved system of language, voice and facial expression, to defuse a threatening situation via the most modern part of the vagus nerve. If that doesn't work, the fight/flight response of the sympathetic nervous system takes over, and if that fails too then the brainstem, via the reptilian vagus, pulls the plugs on the frontal cortex, and possibly on consciousness too, with the freeze/faint response.

One way to think about it is to see the nervous system as the body's security service, with consciousness as the president, or to use an embodied metaphor, the 'head of state'. If the people in dark suits and earpieces need to exercise a little crowd control, they will do it first by polite but firm words, facial expressions and gestures. This is the Social Engagement System at work. But if they sense any real danger, they will immediately hustle the president away in the equivalent of a fight/flight response. If they really think an attack is unavoidable, then the president is pushed unceremoniously to the ground while the Secret Service agents pile on top protectively – the equivalent of a freeze/faint response. According to Porges, the nervous system has this same hierarchy in the way it deals with perceived threats to the bodymind. The first response is usually to try to 'talk down' an aggressor. If this doesn't work, then fight/flight will be the default response, flooding the heart and muscles with the nerve signals and hormones needed for a sudden surge of action. Fainting is the most extreme response, the so-called 'vaso-vagal attack' when the heart rate slows and blood pressure plummets so dramatically that insufficient oxygen reaches the brain and consciousness disappears altogether.

HIS OWN MEDICINE

In fact Porges tells a story of how he experienced this himself. Having spent decades of his career in a multidisciplinary search to understand the different, and apparently contradictory, functions of the vagus nerve, he found himself one day about to undergo an fMRI scan as a diagnostic procedure for a health problem of his own. With colleagues who regularly used the technology in their research, he was intrigued by the prospect of experiencing a scan from the patient's point of view. So imagine his surprise when, as the machine began to slide him head-first into its narrow, noisy interior, with his body deliberately immobilised, he had only got in up to his eyes before he began to feel so uncomfortable that he had to come out again and have a glass of water. On the second attempt, by the time he was in up to his nose he realised that if he went in any further it would trigger a full-scale panic attack. By mutual agreement, he and his medical colleagues stopped the process completely.

Intellectually, Porges was astonished that his nervous system should react in this way to a medical procedure that, ironically, had contributed much to his own research. He now tells the story on the conference circuit to emphasise the point (which is crucial to remember when we use Clean Language) that there is no way to tell just what the bodymind will decide constitutes danger, or what might trigger a fight/flight or freeze/faint response.

'KILL THIS GIRL'

There are three more fs to add to the famous four of fight, flight, freeze and faint. One is for 'fury'. In a parallel but more terrifying experience, Porges' close colleague Peter Levine, after four decades researching how animals and humans respond to trauma, was crossing the road one day when he was hit by a car so hard that his body bounced off the windscreen. In the riveting opening chapter of his book *In an Unspoken Voice* (2010), he describes himself experiencing all the stages of trauma he had studied for so many years: the shaking of his body, the micro-movements of his limbs attempting to complete the protective reflex movements the impact had caused, and also the raw emotional fury, the desire 'to kill this girl' who had so nearly killed him. This kind of rage may be close to the surface day to day in trauma survivors or it may be the most suppressed aspect of the whole traumatic event. If we can acknowledge it and allow it to be experienced as an authentic emotion, then we are likely to find, as Peter Levine did with the help of the paramedic taking him to hospital, that the more modern, myelinated vagus automatically begins to reassert itself, regulating heart rate and blood pressure to bring the person back to a conscious, stable, conversational state.

The other two 'f' words are 'fun' and 'flow'. The fight/flight response is not just there to save us from danger; it is also part of that essential social activity known as play. Physical play, whether sporting or sexual, involves both the adrenal excitement of the sympathetic nervous system and the social engagement of the vagus nerve at the same time. As Porges points out, if dogs involved in fight-play make face-to-face contact after an accidental injury, play will continue. If not, it can quickly turn into a real fight/flight struggle. Thus the Social Engagement System can make all the difference, for example, on the soccer pitch after a hard tackle brings a player painfully to the ground, or outside a club late at night, when a small incident may dissolve in friendly banter or suddenly turn into a murderous attack. In team sports, in business and in family life, we constantly need that highly evolved system and its vagal pathways to help us temper aggression into playful social engagement.

THREE KEY LEARNINGS

Although the polyvagal theory is based on 40 years of research by Porges, it is still a theory, a work in progress. But it seems to be a theory that works and is becoming increasingly popular among psychotherapists, so what can it teach us about how to use Clean Language in bodywork?

FEEL IT, SPEAK IT

The first key point is that the same nerve network that connects us to our visceral sensations also regulates our ability to articulate them. When someone says, 'My heart was in my mouth,' they are offering you a perfect metaphor for how the vagus nerve can either help or hinder our ability to communicate our feelings. A good way to think about this is just to bring your attention to your tongue for a moment. This unique muscle links lungs and larynx to words and speech. Any rigidity in the tongue reflects a rigidity in our ability to let communication flow between body, brain and other people. Knowing how closely connected one part of the vagus nerve is with hearing and speech, and how at the same time, via another part of it, the brainstem can flip us from feeling comfortable and coherent to chaotic and clueless, we begin to understand why it's so important for the therapist to be sensitive to the subtle verbal and non-verbal signals that show just where the client is in relation to the three possible kinds of response: relaxed, aroused or frozen. Understanding the vagus nerve's multiple pathways and functions means we are better able to help clients to stay calmly present with alarming or potentially overwhelming sensations, and better able to use Clean questions to help them find words for those sensations.

When we ask Clean questions we need to notice the subtle hints and early signs of a habitual fight/flight or freeze/faint response, in facial expression, voice tone and breathing. Porges' work reminds us to stay as 'Clean' as we can with our questions, because *you never know* what significance a client may attach to their own words, or indeed to yours. For someone on the autistic spectrum your attempt to make eye contact may seem like a direct threat; for someone trying to deal with the trauma of sexual abuse, your suggestion that they relax their pelvic floor muscles may trigger a panic attack. We never know when the president's bodyguards may instinctively react, or over-react, to some real or imagined danger.

MAMMAL TO MAMMAL

The second key point is to remember that we are mammals, social beings finely tuned to each other's non-verbal signals, and living in a web in which we are unconsciously influencing each other all the time. This is amplified by the 'field' we co-create with our clients in the highly focused atmosphere of a therapy session. Because

Clean questions can take us so deeply into unknown territory with such surprising speed, clients need to know that the person who is there with them is safe to do this with that you the practitioner are comfortable, steady and rooted in your own somatic self, and paying close attention to that steady flow of information about your own internal state that comes to you via the vagus.

LET THE CLIENT TAKE CONTROL

The third key point brings us back to one of the core principles of Clean Language – that as far as possible the client stays in control of their own experience. When strong feelings arise, always let them know they can pause or stop at any time, and make sure you have their permission before asking another question. Use language that invites rather than instructs; ask questions rather than giving commands. In other words, stay as Clean as you can – never assuming you know what is going on for your client or what is best for them. Unless your client really does go into an uncontrolled traumatic response (in which case use eye contact, voice and touch to reassure them until they have calmed down), all they need from you is the stable and compassionate presence of a fellow mammal. When you use Clean Language in this way, you enormously enhance not only the trust the client has in you but also, and more important, their trust that they can listen to their own body and its peculiar ways of communicating what it knows.

So now we've seen how the bodymind can hold information as a 'felt sense' and how that information can either be locked into the tissues by trauma, or find its way via the vagus nerve up through the brainstem and into consciousness. Like the hero of a good thriller, it has survived the original trauma, escaped from its captors and now seems to have arrived back at headquarters for debriefing. But in good thrillers, headquarters are never what they seem. Your own brain can be a treacherous place, where it can be hard to know who's on your side, or indeed, whose side you're on.

For the final part of our exploration of how words and feelings interact, let's look at the relationship between the two sides of our brain and how it constructs our lived reality.

∽ 18 ∽

THE DIVIDED BRAIN

So what happens to 'felt sense' and the many subtle things we may be aware of *through* the body when they finally make their way up to the brain? How does the brain make sense of them, and why is it often so hard to trust or even listen to the kind of information the body has to offer? Could it be something about how the brain connects with the body – something about the brain itself?

There are various ways to look at the brain, all of them subject to some degree of debate among neuroscientists. First there is the 'triune brain', the vertical evolutionary view from brainstem to cortex. Second, there are important differences between what the front, middle and rear parts of the brain do. Then if you view the brain from the front as a kind of vertical sandwich, there are distinctions between what the two sides do (the bread) compared to the middle (the filling). More controversially but inevitably, there are differences between the male and female brain. But by far the most obvious and startling fact about the brain, be it male or female, human or animal, is that it is divided into two almost completely separate halves, and those two hemispheres seem to relate to the body in very different ways.

For centuries, medical science accumulated anecdotal evidence that there might be differences between the two sides of the brain, largely through studying the effects of severe head injuries and strokes. But the idea that the two sides of the brain have completely different job descriptions (that the left brain is 'verbal' and 'logical' while the right brain is 'intuitive' and 'creative') became suddenly popular in the 1960s following research into the effects of split brain surgery for people suffering from chronic epileptic fits. By severing the corpus callosum – nerve fibres that connect the two hemispheres – doctors were able to prevent these fits, and when psychologists did research into how people experienced the world when the communication between the two sides of the brain was so severely reduced, they did indeed find significant differences between what each hemisphere did when left to its own devices.

More recently, with the vastly increased ability to study human brains in action which neuro-imaging technology has made possible, neuroscientists have continued to find many examples of what they call 'hemispheric asymmetry'. But what neuro-imaging has also shown is that almost everything we do involves simultaneous activity on *both* sides of the brain. Confronted by this paradox, and perhaps keen to distance the serious business of neuroscience from the crude 'left brain/right brain' caricature that had become so embedded in popular culture, neuroscientists continued to map the 'what' of hemispherical difference but tended to avoid asking the bigger questions of how or why the two sides of the brain could be so separate and why that separation has increased rather than decreased over the course of human evolution.

So the third mind/body pioneer I would like to introduce you to is the psychiatrist Dr Iain McGilchrist, one of the few people who continued to ask, when most neuroscientists considered the subject a dead end, how this fact that our brains are divided in two influences the way we *experience* the world (including our own bodies) and affects how we then try to *shape* that world.

Twenty years in the writing, his book *The Master and his Emissary* (McGilchrist 2010)1 is an extraordinary multidisciplinary feat of scholarship and insight. While it has been greeted with approval, much of it lavish, by leading authorities in the field, it is still in the early stages of being digested by mainstream neuroscience and the many other disciplines it has implications for, including our own field of bodywork therapy.

A DIFFERENCE OF VALUES

McGilchrist's essential thesis is that the two sides of our brain not only absorb and process information in significantly different ways, but attach different values to that information and how to use it in the world. His book is the story of a relationship, at once both cooperative and competitive, in which each side needs the other's help to be able to do its own job fully, but while one side – the right hemisphere – knows this, the left side believes that it can manage perfectly well on its own.

Using clinical cases of how trauma, lesions, tumours and strokes affect brain function, as well as the revelations of modern neuro-imaging, McGilchrist meticulously assembles the most in-depth analysis in the literature of neuroscience of what we know (so far) about the differences between the two sides of the brain. While both hemispheres are intimately involved in almost every aspect of mental activity, they seem to have very different priorities. The right side of our brain is better at attuning to awareness in the moment, to being open to new experience, to empathy, relationship, cooperation and – crucially for our purposes – to what the body knows. Meanwhile, the left side of the brain is more attuned to past and future, and is interested in one's own individual needs rather than cooperating with others (see figure on page 168). The left hemisphere finds it hard to acknowledge information that conflicts with what it already knows, and – again crucial from the mind/body therapist's point of view – sees the body more as a machine than an organism and has an inherent distrust of 'gut feelings', of the complex embodied kind of knowing which Gendlin calls 'felt sense'.

Put like this it is easy to see the right hemisphere as the good side and the left hemisphere as the villain. In the table below, the often-opposing values and attributes of the two sides might seem to confirm this, but this competition between the two hemispheres, McGilchrist suggests, is actually healthy, like the Chinese idea of Yin and Yang. Information is constantly flowing back and forth between the two sides, not only through the corpus callosum but also through the sub-cortical connections that they share, each side absorbing information from the body and the external world in its own way, doing its best to inhibit some aspects of the opposite hemisphere's reality in order to do its own job properly, while sampling moment to moment something of what the other side is doing.

THE DIFFERENT PRIORITIES OF THE LEFT AND RIGHT HEMISPHERES OF THE BRAIN

Left hemisphere	Right hemisphere
Theory	Facts
Concepts	Phenomena
Competition	Cooperation
Meaning of words	Tone and expression
Static, fixed	Movement in time and space
Anger	Other emotions
Own needs	Needs of wider group
Focused vision	Peripheral vision
Literal	Understands metaphor
Mechanical	Organic
Simple rhythm	Music and complex rhythm
Virtual	Rooted in bodily experience
Single meanings	Ambiguity

Certainty	Paradox
Isolated pieces of information	Entity as a whole and in context
Detached observation	Openness to Other
What fits the pattern?	What doesn't fit the pattern?
Recognises only what it knows	Open to what's new
Reductionist	Holistic
Theoretical	Pragmatic
Utilitarian	Aesthetic
Reaching to grasp	Holding
Right hand	Left hand
Clear categories	Subtle differences
Dominates in adult	Dominates age 0–4 years
Reads mouth	Reads eyes
Powerful operator	Patient recipient
Books, films, video games	Real life
Doesn't know it needs RH	Knows it needs LH
Individual identity	Individual as part of a group
English – sounds as phonic building blocks	Chinese – sounds depend on tonality and context
Horizontal	Vertical
Left to right	Right to left
Denial	Taking too much responsibility
Future-directed	In the moment
Focus of attention	Intensity of attention
Liberty, equality as abstract principles	How people really behave
Flat, two-dimensional	Depth, three-dimensional
Schematic	Complex
Simple shapes	Natural shapes
Names of body parts	Map of body parts
Best in routine situations	Best in new situations

Compiled by Nick Pole based on information from McGilchrist (2010).

This division of labour between the hemispheres, which humans share with all other mammals and birds, seems to have emerged in response to one of the most basic problems of survival – how to stay focused on hunting for one's own food while being alert enough to avoid becoming someone else's. The left hemisphere excels at finding the food – at tasks which demand highly focused attention and the ability to recognise and sort between categories of things it has already learned, the edible and the poisonous, for example. Meanwhile, the right hemisphere is far better at maintaining a wide horizon of awareness, at being open to anything, known or unknown, which may suddenly appear as a potential threat.

The right hemisphere's ability to be so open to the outside world seems to have developed, as mammals evolved, into a relational ability to be aware of and open to the existence of the 'other' and specifically to cuddle, cradle or connect with a mate, a newborn or another member of the group. This 'betweenness', as McGilchrist calls it (2010, p.95), is a natural attribute of the right hemisphere, well documented for example in studies of neural activity in mothers and babies. The right hemisphere is the first to develop in the womb, and is the one best suited for the way newborns learn to communicate, through touch, facial expression and non-verbal sound.

Then around the age of six months, the ability to reach out and grasp things develops at the same time as the urge to reach out verbally by trying to form specific sounds and, later, actual words. McGilchrist emphasises how closely these two activities are associated in the brain. The area for processing the basic content and meaning of verbal speech is in the left hemisphere next to the area which controls grasping movements of the right hand, the hand which for most people is dominant in manipulating and controlling the world around them. The bodywork therapist Bill Palmer suggests that this link between the thumb and index finger of the right hand and the speech centre in the brain originated because the first language was probably sign language, accompanied by grunts (Palmer 1995, p.10). Whatever the origin, metaphor reveals how close this connection is: the word 'grasp' can apply as much to ideas as to material objects, and the same metaphor is at work whenever I ask if you 'get' what I mean. As we learn how the fingers and thumb of the right hand allow us to manipulate objects with great precision, so we learn how words give us that precise ability to make things happen inside other people's heads.

Meanwhile, the right hemisphere, perhaps because it is responsible for two functions essential to survival – the wide-open alertness to the outside world and the ability of mother and baby to communicate – is more intuitively connected with the body than the left hemisphere is. While each side of the brain has its own motor and sensory cortex connecting it to the *opposite* side of the body, McGilchrist points out that the right hemisphere has the more sophisticated image of the body and what it's doing; not just a visual image but 'a sense of the body as a coherent, living (and lived) whole' (Rowson and McGilchrist 2013).

Perhaps also because of its vital role in fostering communication between mother and child, the right hemisphere's sense of relationship is based on empathy and cooperation, while the left hemisphere thinks of relationship as a means to an end, a way of influencing people and things to achieve particular goals. Without the left hemisphere we would live in a world of pure awareness, in which nothing ever got done. In her book *My Stroke of Insight* (2008b) and in her TED talk online (2008a), neuroscientist Jill Bolte Taylor brilliantly describes both the enlightenment and the frustration of this state of being, which she experienced when she suffered a massive left-hemisphere stroke. Amazed by her blazing, present-moment sense of oneness with everything around her, she realised at the same time that she had lost the ability to speak or understand speech. What most of us are more familiar with – and this is a crucial part of McGilchrist's argument – is life lived mainly from the left brain, a world of *perpetual* doing, goal-oriented and future-focused, with only the barest sense of relationship with others or ourselves.

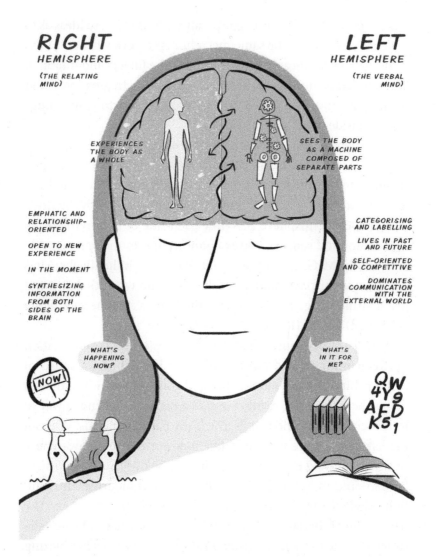

The divided brain

Just as different departments in an organisation can develop very different values and ways of doing things, so have the two sides of our brains. But in an organisation there is a CEO, someone who can listen to both sides, who can bring in consultants to help resolve conflicts, and the CEO has an office and a name. The fascinating thing about the brain is that no one knows yet, in any scientific sense, where to find the CEO. The ability to observe one's own mind in action, to notice those sudden moments or habitual contexts in which we find ourselves too much in the left or the right side of the brain, seems to emerge somehow from the systemic interaction of both hemispheres with the sub-cortical parts of the brain and perhaps, as we discover in both meditation and Focusing, from the ability of the brain to reconnect with the body.

SYNTHESISING EXPERIENCE INTO KNOWING

'Life can certainly have meaning without books,' says McGilchrist, 'but books cannot have meaning without life' (2010, p.195), making absolutely clear in one sentence what he calls the 'primacy' of the right hemisphere. The fundamental difference between the two hemispheres, he says, is that the right brain is like someone who learns about life by *living* it, while the left brain is like someone who can only learn about life from *reading* about it (the way I tried to do as a painfully shy teenager). But McGilchrist himself is a man who has acquired a vast wealth of knowledge from books, and his appreciation for the left hemisphere is evident in the model he suggests to describe what happens when the two hemispheres are working well together. The right hemisphere's first job is to synthesise sensory in-the-moment information about what is happening and then to send that across to be analysed in terms of all the labels and categories, past associations and future possibilities that the left hemisphere uses to process experience, above all to turn raw sensory data into *words*.

Once understood in this way, the information is then returned to the right hemisphere to do its second, more sophisticated job, which is to apply that analysis of its original sensory data in a practical way to the ever-changing complexity of the living world. The analogy makes it very clear how much the right hemisphere depends on the left. As McGilchrist puts it, what we read in books (left hemisphere) comes from the lived experience of their authors (right hemisphere), but when we read these books, it 'not only *adds* to life, but genuinely goes back into life and *transforms* it' (2010, p.196). This takes place moment to moment, but also over the longer term in the fulfilment of any particular project or task. The French film director Robert Bresson gives a beautiful example of this in his *Notes on Cinematography* (1977, p.7):

> My movie is born first in my head, dies on paper; is resuscitated by the living persons and real objects I use, which are killed on film but, placed in a certain order and projected on to a screen, come to life again like flowers in water.

In terms of how the left and right hemispheres work, Bresson's sense that his movie is 'born first in my head' refers to the way inspiration pops into consciousness via the right hemisphere; then in writing it down, the left hemisphere is dominant; it 'dies on paper' – in other words, as a script it loses the sense of direct connection to lived experience which only the right hemisphere provides. This is 'resuscitated by the living persons and real objects I use' – the moment-to-moment experience of actually shooting the film, in which the right hemisphere is constantly alive and alert. These real people and objects 'are killed on film', trapped frame by frame on celluloid to be manipulated in the editing room, but 'placed in a certain order and projected on to a screen, come to life again like flowers in water'. Notice the metaphor. Bresson's 'flowers in water' is his way of describing the power of cinema to hold us in the moment, to suspend our left-brain disbelief, to identify with people we have never met and feel the emotions they are feeling. At the same time, of course, we are also thinking, 'Do I believe this?', 'How did they shoot that?' and 'What other films have I seen her in?' – questions that keep the left hemisphere occupied while the right brain enjoys one of its particular specialities, the power of story-telling.

Another way to think about it might be a tennis player, who needs the right hemisphere's moment-to-moment awareness of the other player's moves and of the flight of the ball as it comes across the net, while at the same time using a left-hemisphere library of what kind of moves their opponent might make and all the ways the ball could behave, as well as an understanding of what kind of point is being played, at what stage in the match, and so on. This information then goes back to the right brain, which specialises in spatial awareness and movement of the body, whose higher-level task is now to coordinate eyes, muscles, racquet and energy either to conjure an amazing volley or perhaps to let the ball go because the risk or the effort would not be worth the point.

WHOLE BRAIN THINKING

When both hemispheres are working well together, we have 'whole brain thinking' – the kind of thinking that includes bodily awareness and felt sense as valid information (see figure on page 174). When this happens for someone as I ask them Clean questions, I feel that something has indeed 'come to life', as they spontaneously begin to move from a predominantly left-hemisphere frame of mind, talking only in terms of the labels and the history which they or the medical professionals may have given their problem, and start to shift into an awareness of how they are right now, in the moment, exploring the 'Where…?', the 'What kind of…?' and the 'Anything else…?' of what they're experiencing, and noticing as they do that the bodymind nearly always begins to respond in some way to having this kind of attention paid to it.

One crucial thing that is coming to life in these moments is the left hemisphere's willingness to learn something new. While it thinks mainly in terms of abstract labels, maps and categories and (like an old-fashioned librarian), can get easily irritated by the arrival of new information which doesn't fit into its meticulously catalogued world, it must be able to rise to the challenge of adding categories and maps to its already extensive collection, otherwise we would never learn anything new. Just as the field of language teaching now uses multi-sensory input to make it easier for the left hemisphere to embed the phrases of a foreign 'tongue', so Clean questions bring a heightened awareness and sense of challenge to the left hemisphere. It learns that communication is actually possible with the 'dark territories' of the body, of pain, of emotional confusion and subtle felt sense, and looks for ways to understand these things in the only way it knows how – by finding words that fit them.

THE RIGHT HEMISPHERE KNOWS BUT CAN'T SAY

Virginia Woolf knew this intuitively and for a very good reason. A victim of childhood sexual abuse by an older half-brother, she was brought up by parents who valued her left-hemisphere skills with language and the written word far more than they valued the simple warmth of human relationship. Suffering from illness and depression throughout her adult life, she knew more than most people about the difficulty of finding words for interior pain. In an essay, *On Being Ill*, she wrote:

> Let a sufferer try to describe a pain in his head to a doctor and language at once runs dry. There is nothing ready made for him. He is forced to coin words himself, and, taking his pain in one hand, and a lump of pure sound in the other...so to crush them together that a brand new word in the end drops out. Probably it will be something laughable. (2002, p.7)

Here Woolf captures the right hemisphere's urgent, inarticulate need to shape its sensations and impressions into communicable form. Invariably, as Woolf points out (probably unconsciously) it does it first non-verbally, with gesture – the movement of the two hands – but like a traveller who cannot speak the local language, there is still the frustrated urge to find the right words; and the left hemisphere's characteristic response when it hears something unintelligible, something other than its own language, is to find it 'laughable'.

There is no more powerful or poignant example of this than the story of the young Helen Keller, born in 1880 in Alabama and rendered deaf, blind and mute by illness at the age of 19 months. After five years of terrible frustration, living as 'less than an animal' (as she later described it) in a wordless world of pure sensation, her desperate parents hired Anne Sullivan, a partially sighted teacher from Boston. The film *The Miracle Worker* vividly depicts Sullivan's compassionate and ruthless determination to discipline this feral bundle of rage enough to teach her how to spell words with her hands. After several weeks, though she learns many, she still has no idea what these odd movements of her hands are supposed to mean. Then one day at the water pump the little girl discovers that the letters her teacher is spelling on her palm are the *name* of the liquid flow she can feel as she holds her other hand under the spout. In the film you can see Sullivan (played by Anne Bancroft, who won an Oscar for the role) watching Helen's moment of awakening in amazement. 'Water!! That word startled my soul, and it awoke,' Keller later wrote. 'Until that day my mind had been like a darkened chamber, waiting for words to enter and light the lamp, which is thought' (Keller 1909/2009, p.120).

To watch Helen's epiphany (easily done on YouTube) is a great way to remind yourself that all those moments of blankness, bafflement and silent confusion that your clients may experience when they hear your Clean questions are signs that their left hemisphere is doing its best to give a *name* to whatever the right hemisphere may be wordlessly presenting to it. It is a great reminder too that the right hemisphere *knows* how much it needs the left, while the left hemisphere, wrapped up in the virtual reality of its concepts, theories and categories, needs constantly to be reminded of the importance of attending to its partner on the right.

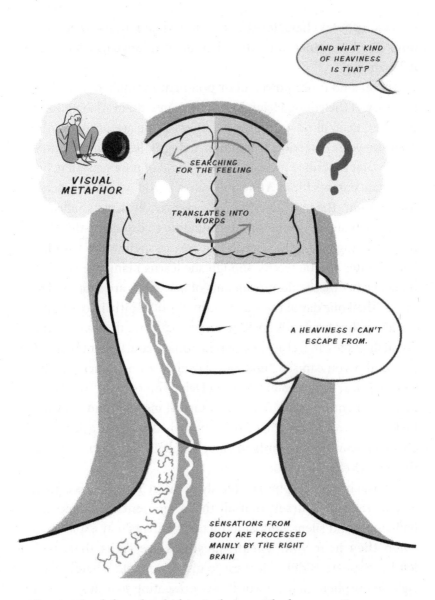

Connecting left and right hemispheres with clean questions

SO WHAT DOES IT ALL MEAN FOR
MIND/BODY THERAPY?

If your client seems stuck as they try to answer your Clean question, it is almost certainly because they are still struggling with this right-to-left process. For example, the right hemisphere may be offering a metaphorical image of a thick fog, but as far as the left hemisphere knows, the doctor said it was 'depression' and that's all there is to it. When a client's thinking becomes symptom bound, it's a sign that they are stuck in this left-hemisphere kind of thinking, where everything is experienced in terms of what is already known – where news of difference is welcome only if it can be connected in some way to the labels and categories that are already there. Watch your client's eye movements, attend to their silences and notice their gestures and body language as they try to come up with words that fit their feelings, since these are all signs that left and right hemispheres are doing their best to work together to come up with an intelligible answer to your Clean question.

Be patient with the left hemisphere's habit of ignoring the non-verbal information that the right hemisphere is offering it. It has a managerial mind-set and sees no value in things that cannot be accurately measured or precisely described, and has a natural tendency to say 'No' when you ask questions like, '**And is there anything else about** that pain in your shoulder?' And when something does come in words, the left hemisphere will often, as Virginia Woolf pointed out, find those words 'laughable' and try to distance itself from what it is about to say with phrases you will hear again and again like 'This sounds silly...' or 'I don't know where this is coming from but...' Learn to recognise these phrases as a sign that successful communication between the two hemispheres has begun!

A WRITER'S FEAR OF HIS BODY

Clean questions are one way we can bring the client to the edge of their verbally defined world and inspire curiosity about what lies beyond. This vital step in healing is memorably described by the writer Tim Parks, who was afflicted in his 50s by agonising pelvic pains. Used to treating his body in a typically left-hemisphere way, as a machine designed essentially for connecting his mind to the physical world, he explored every possible medical treatment but without success. Intensely sceptical of alternative therapies, in desperation he began to experiment with a particular way of bringing mindful awareness to his own symptoms, and to his surprise he found some relief. These meditative exercises involved a different kind of concentration – in fact a different kind of *thought* – from anything that, as a professional writer and translator, he was used to. In his book *Teach Us to Sit Still* (Parks 2010, p.172), he describes how he:

> never really appreciated that there could be hard mental work that *did not involve words*, work for which, on the contrary, words might prove an obstacle... For decades now, I realized, all purposeful mental activity for me had been linguistic: writing, thinking, reasoning, teaching, talking... Everything had to be lived through language or it wasn't lived at all, to the point that I hadn't really *seen* a painting or a film (or a game of football for that matter) until I had thought about it in words, or preferably talked about it, or better still written about it... Then I *possessed* it.

That honest word 'possessed' is so important in understanding the left hemisphere's attitude to the world. By naming things, categorising them and filing them away in its vast virtual library it has a sense, if not of owning them, at least of being able to make use of them as tools for extending its control over the external world. And this attitude extends to the body it lives in. When parts of the body go wrong, the left hemisphere gets annoyed with them and looks for ways to fix them as quickly as possible. The sense of detachment that it has from its own malfunctioning parts is real – lacking the right hemisphere's richer web of somatic connection, the left hemisphere thinks about its own body the way it thinks about everything else, as something which is important only insofar as it can help it get on with that great and ongoing 'to do' list which, over in the right hemisphere, is known as life.

A CLEAN RELATIONSHIP BETWEEN LEFT AND RIGHT

One reason Clean questions can help to weave left and right hemispheres together is that they use an apparently clear and logical kind of language that appeals to the left hemisphere. But each Clean question about somatic experience is an invitation to the left hemisphere to remember that it does after all need the right hemisphere to be able to come up with an answer to what is happening in the body right now. And as clients learn how to ask themselves Clean questions, perhaps they are already beginning to change their own neural patterning, developing more sensitive networks of awareness, sensation and thought between these two sides of the brain.

Also, as you use Clean questions and the emergent wisdom that they cultivate in us, you are not just introducing the left hemisphere to the body (via the right hemisphere) you are also inviting your client to develop a more cooperative, empathic attitude to their whole mind/brain/body, as many mindfulness-based approaches encourage us to do. 'Be kinder to yourself,' is not always a helpful suggestion to make directly to your client if, for example, they are suffering from depression or anxiety, when being kind to oneself is actually one of the hardest things to do. But when the suggestion is made indirectly through Clean questions, ones which simply invite the client to bring focused and attentive curiosity to their own body, and each question is based not on some therapeutic concept but on the exact words the client just said, then the left hemisphere necessarily begins to find itself in a dialogue with the right, where these qualities of empathy and kindness naturally reside.

Of course, it's also important for you as the practitioner to *embody* these qualities as part of that invitation, in your intention, posture, face and tone of voice. As Alan Schore, another profoundly influential figure in the integration of neuroscience and therapy, has pointed out, 'Just as the left brain communicates its states to other left brains via conscious linguistic behaviours, so the right non-verbally communicates its unconscious states to other right brains that are tuned to receive these communications' (2010, p.184). In this way, though the minds of both client and practitioner may keep wandering into the left hemisphere's verbal domain, Clean Language reminds us to come back to a whole-brain, whole-body way for client and practitioner to be present with themselves and each other.

PART 3
THE PRACTICE

3.1 INTRODUCTION

∼

I'm in Amsterdam with my friend and colleague, Peter den Dekker, qi gong teacher and author of *The Dynamics of Standing Still* (2010), an innovative introduction to 'Zhan Zhuang', the 'Standing like a Tree' style of qi gong. We're watching a group of his students working together in groups of three as I introduce them to Clean Language. Some are bodywork therapists, some are not, and I'm wondering how Clean Language might help them. A woman calls me over; she seems to have got stuck. Her face is set in a heavy frown, and she says that she doesn't think the Clean questions will work for her the way they worked for me when I demonstrated the process earlier. Her problem seems to be with the Outcome question, so I ask her what she would like to have happen. She says:

 – To have a back massage.

And what would that be like, *to have a back massage?*

She thinks for a moment.

 – No, actually I want an arm resting across the top of my shoulders.

And what would that be like, an arm resting across the top of your shoulders?
- Supportive (her frown has begun to soften slightly).

And is there anything else about supportive?
- It's warm and comfortable.

And when an arm across the top of your shoulders is supportive and warm and comfortable, then what happens?
- Then I relax.

And is there anything else about relax?
- (She puts a hand on the centre of her chest) Then I feel more in touch with myself here.

Now her frown has gone, replaced by a look of gentle concentration. I slip out of Clean Language, to ask if she's aware that there is much more colour in her face now. She breaks into a smile – so do I – saying that, no, she hadn't realised that, but now she can feel it. And as she feels it, she says, she notices the warm feeling spreading through her shoulders, and a sense that they are already more relaxed.

This woman is an experienced bodywork therapist, but says she's 'amazed' at how quickly her body has responded to just a few simple questions – amazed that she didn't actually need a back massage or an arm resting on her shoulders to feel so different and so in touch with herself. Imagine if she had come to you for a bodywork session, how much more responsive to your techniques she might be after those few questions, compared to that frowning place she started from.

This woman's experience encapsulates what this book is all about: how readily the bodymind responds when you communicate with it in language it can understand. Clean questions make sense to the bodymind and are by nature an invitation for the two sides of the brain to work together. They invite the left hemisphere to recognise that it needs the right hemisphere's embodied intelligence, and at the same time they help the right hemisphere appreciate that language has a healing power of its own.

~ **19** ~

HOW TO STRUCTURE A SESSION

What first drew me to Clean Language was a sense that somehow it mirrored very closely the principles of my Japanese teacher's way of working with touch: the profound respect for the client's space and boundaries, starting where the client is at, moving at their pace and allowing them to lead the way – these are all inherent in the Chinese concept of 'Wu Wei', of doing 'Non-doing', of minimal intervention, of following the client's flow without imposing on it.

As I learned more about Clean Language, I realised that the two approaches do indeed share some common principles, even though they start from very different places. Shiatsu is rooted in traditional Japanese bodywork and culture, while Clean Language owes much to modern systems theory – the study of how complex systems like living organisms or weather patterns or the World Wide Web function and evolve in response to what goes on within them and around them. But despite systems theory's modern origins, in a way it is simply a beautiful update of the ancient Taoist principles from which China's traditional forms of both healing and the martial arts evolved. In both, each individual living being is seen as a complex of interacting functions, separate from and at the same time inseparably part of the larger systems that sustain it. From the energy patterns of our own individual bodymind to the eco-system of the planet as a whole, we are all part of what Ted Kaptchuk in his pioneering book *Chinese Medicine* (1983) called, 'the web that has no weaver'.

When applied to mind/body therapy, both approaches suggest to me a way of working based on these five principles:

1. Create an empty, listening space between you and the client.

2. Interfere as little as possible with what arises for the client in this space.

3. Work only with what the client offers you (both consciously and unconsciously, through words, gestures, movements and energy).

4. Use the simplest possible techniques.

5. Trust that somewhere inside, the client already knows what they really need and is looking for a way to show you how to help them take the next step to finding it.

When you take this approach, the challenge is in that word 'Trust' – this is what underlies the whole concept of 'Non-doing'. The more you trust, the less you do. As Peter Itin puts it in *Shiatsu als Therapie* (2007, p.189):

> As the therapist, my inner attitude during the dialogue is, 'Everything you need to know is already there, but it won't appear from your conceptual mind.' This relieves me of having to be the omniscient counsellor, and my only responsibility is to create an appropriate 'vessel' through which the client's inner knowing can come.[1]

---

1 Thanks to Verna Schwalm for translating parts of this book for me.

FROM PRINCIPLES TO PRACTICE

Because Clean Language can be so effective at working through the protective layers we normally wrap ourselves in, it requires a lot from us as practitioners, question by question, always to be one step ahead in our willingness to accept, be present with and curious about whatever comes up, however much it may trigger the natural reactions that we are humanly prone to. Of course there will be judgements, presuppositions and prejudices arising for us all the time – minds do that – but if we simply remain grounded, mindful and present, ready to listen and respond in an embodied way, then we create the mental space we need to keep track of the complex internal landscape our client is exploring. This could be said of many kinds of therapy but Clean Language seems particularly effective at getting to the core of an issue rapidly while at the same time making it clear to the client that it is their own words and gestures that have got them into that landscape.

In this third part of the book we'll look at how to put these basic principles into action, how they work in clinical practice and what to do when they don't. Except for one, the case studies that make up Part 3 all come from my own practice with clients and my own way of working, mixing Clean Language with meridian-based bodywork based on notions like Yin and Yang and the Five Elements of traditional Chinese medicine. Since these ideas may be very different from yours, not only in terms of the techniques you use but also in terms of basic philosophy and principles, I have focused mainly on how the Clean Language dialogues in each case study create their own shifts for the client in both body and mind. Sometimes I include details of the bodywork part of the sessions when there is a clear connection with what we've already achieved with our Clean dialogue, but I have tried to keep the jargon of my own shiatsu-based approach to a minimum. I've also included interviews with several different bodywork and movement therapists, explaining the various ways they use Clean Language with their clients and students, in the hope that no matter how much my own methods may differ from yours, you can find some help and guidance there.

In line with current practice in preserving confidentiality, not only have identifying details been changed – most of these case studies are not transcripts of one actual session but integrate my experiences of working with two or more different clients, each of whom has read a transcript of their session and given me permission to use it. One exception to this is 'The Root of the Problem that Causes the Pain', which is a transcript of a workshop demonstration in which the person I was working with read the transcript and gave her full permission to use it.

For some reason, a lot of people who start learning Clean Language develop quite rigid ideas about keeping their dialogue completely 'Clean', thinking that they're getting it wrong if they include any other kind of question. In Chapter 30, we'll look at when it might be better to let go of Clean questions (and why), and at some alternative forms of 'facilitative language' which can have an equal effect if your client is not responding well to your attempts to be Clean. Here in Part 3, don't be surprised if you find me sometimes using language which is not completely Clean. It is there to show you how I might combine Clean Language with other approaches, depending on what seems appropriate for the client.

I've tried to write the case studies as 'good stories', otherwise you probably wouldn't read them. And most of them end successfully, one or two spectacularly so, since you probably wouldn't want to try Clean Language with your own clients if they didn't. But I don't want to imply that I get such results with every client. You may well be a better bodywork therapist than I am and get similar results without Clean Language, or any kind of language at all. My point is simply that by using Clean Language I am making sure the client is more involved in, if not actually leading, a collaborative process.

Neither do I want to imply that every client takes to the Clean approach as well as the clients in these stories do. Every client is different, and if you are starting out with Clean Language, it's probably best not to inflict it on clients who clearly aren't comfortable with it. But the more experience you get with Clean questions, the better you will be at working out exactly what's right for each person you work with.

Finally, at the end of each case study I have included some brief comments to emphasise the learning points and to help you make sense of the sometimes confusing twists and turns that most Clean sessions contain. If, however, you are the kind of bodyworker (very rare, in my experience) who is interested in more abstract analysis of how Clean questions work, with diagrams and flow charts to explain the underlying structures of Clean dialogue, then I can wholeheartedly recommend Marion Way's superb *Clean Approaches for Coaches* (2013). This will give you all those things and more, including an introduction to Clean Language's subtle and sophisticated big sister – Symbolic Modelling – the approach to working with metaphor landscapes developed from David Grove's work by James Lawley and Penny Tompkins (2000).

AN 8-STEP STRUCTURE FOR A
CLEAN BODYWORK SESSION

A common question that bodywork therapists ask me about using Clean Language is, 'How much time will it take up in the session?' The honest answer is that asking Clean questions and being prepared to go wherever they take you may well mean there is less time for the bodywork. Because I find this a rewarding way to work, I often do sessions lasting about two hours. But some of my shiatsu colleagues use Clean questions far more succinctly than I do and find they actually make the verbal part of the session shorter. Sometimes just a few Clean questions can make a big difference, and having a clear structure in mind about how you use Clean Language during a session will also save time. Here are the eight steps I usually follow when I use Clean Language in my sessions.

1. First, check how Clean your opening question is. 'What brings you here?' implies that they were brought by some

outside force. 'How can I help?' might imply that you're going to fix them. Unless they know the rules of Clean Language, it's too soon to ask, '**What would you like to have happen?**' You need to know where they are before you ask them where they want to go. 'Where would you like to begin?' is a pretty Clean question, so I often start with that. Whatever the response, use as many Clean questions as you can to find out more about it, and how and where it connects with the body, if that is appropriate.

2. Next, ask about their outcome – what would they like to have happen in relation to what they have told you so far? Use Clean questions to help them explore this and don't stop until you notice some kind of bodily shift happening. They haven't really connected with their outcome until it registers somehow in the body.

3. When you have a sense that it's time to start the bodywork, ask your client if that would be okay. If not, continue with Clean questions until it is.

4. When you start the bodywork part of the session, be alert to moments when a Clean question might be helpful, but remember that they may prefer not to talk. They may already have a lot to process as a result of the questions you've already asked, and the bodywork part of the session provides time to let that happen.

5. When the bodywork is done, check how your client is. Remember, language may not come easily to them if they have been very engaged with movement and body sensations, or if your work has left them in a deeply relaxed state. But when they're ready, ask them to recall the original outcome they had before the bodywork began, and what their sense of it is now. Remember they may not be aware of this only as bodily sensations but also as thoughts, sounds, words, imagery, metaphor or movement.

6. Then, if appropriate, ask them to check what sense they have of the original problem. How is that now? Usually it will either have much less charge to it or it will have disappeared completely. That doesn't mean it's gone, just that they're in a much more resourceful place in relation to it now.

7. If appropriate, ask them what they can do next time the problem recurs, if it does. Invite them to rehearse this by reminding them of the problem now that they are in this more relaxed, resourceful state. How would they deal with it now? If they are the kind of client who likes some 'homework', then that is something they can take away to practise.

8. Finally, ask if there's anything else. If not, then ask if that's a good place to finish.

∾ 20 ∾

SORTING OUT THE
RUBIK'S CUBE

Here's an example of how you might adapt that basic structure, according to the way your client actually responds. It's based on a session I did once at the offices of a corporate client where people were coming in for half-hour 'taster' sessions. With this particular client I deliberately used Clean Language to get the best result I could for her in the shortest possible time.

She arrives a few minutes late, apologetic that she's been delayed by a difficult call. I ask if there's anything particular she'd like from the session. She says she doesn't know what it could do for her, because she's never had shiatsu before. I quickly explain the kind of problems it can help with, and ask again if there's anything particular she wants. 'To have more energy,' she replies.

Unlike most people, she's started with a clearly stated outcome. The tightness around her jaw, her slightly narrowed eyes and the tension in her neck and shoulders all suggest that there's a problem in there somewhere. But I understand enough about corporate culture to know that people prefer to talk in terms of outcomes rather than problems. I ask:

And how would that be, *to have more energy?*
- I would be back on track. (She straightens a little in her chair – her body has already started to get involved in the conversation.)

And is there anything else about *back on track?*

She starts to gesture with little twists of her wrists, her hands in front of her solar plexus, palms slightly apart, as if holding something between them. I am fascinated because what she's doing looks identical to a movement from tai chi. At least, that's how I see it. After a while, the words come to explain what these movements mean to her:

- The Rubik's cube would be sorted out.

And when *the Rubik's cube is sorted out,* *that's like what?*

Suddenly, her expression changes, her upper body softens and her eyes gaze out through the window; she is silent for a while and then says:

- It would be like a whole new avenue opening up.

Something has really shifted for her. Her eyes and jaw relax and there is a lightness to her presence that wasn't there before.

Often on these corporate days, people come in, flop down and soak up whatever you can give them before snapping back into work mode and heading out of the door, their minds already back at work, even if in a more relaxed body. This woman seems to be operating at a different level.

I gently mirror her change of posture.

And is there anything else about *a whole new avenue opening up?*

This time she gestures up and down the midline of her body, and says softly:

- Peace…serenity.

I am impressed, even a bit moved. She may think she knows nothing about shiatsu, but her body seems to think differently and is only too keen to make that clear. To my meridian-based way of thinking, the gesture she has just made follows a channel which is known as a 'reservoir of energy' – just what she said she wanted.

Her state has already changed profoundly and her gestures have given me clear indications about the connections she wants the bodywork to make. I ask if that would be a good point to start the treatment, and she lies down on the couch and gets herself comfortable, still very much aware, it seems, of this sense of peace and serenity. Even when time is short, once a client is lying down I always ask them to notice how they're breathing and if there's anything they're aware of that's drawing their attention.

- It feels rather tight around my neck and shoulders.

I ask her where exactly that tight feeling is, where it seems to come from. As I do, my hands are already working with it, around it and into it, feeling the response in her muscles as she does that. She has closed her eyes and I decide not to ask her any more questions for now. I work her lower back, her knees, her feet, and then come back to her neck and ask how it is there now. She keeps her eyes closed, nods slightly and smiles a little. As we get close to finishing, I ask her how she is now.

- My neck feels a lot better. Thank you.

Anything else?

There's a pause, as if she's wondering whether to mention something or not.

- Am I supposed to feel so tired?

Hmm. She wanted more energy and now she's feeling tired. What shall I do? I could ask her about the demands her work is making on her, or say that sometimes that's how the body responds, or ask about her sleep, or how much tea and coffee she drinks. But if her bodymind has decided to let her be tired, it probably has a good reason for that, so let's stay with the Clean approach.

What kind of *tired is that tired?*
- It's a good kind of tired. Like when I wake up in my yoga class and realise I've been asleep.

And is there anything else about *that good kind of tired?*
- It's okay. It's how I get more energy.

She has remembered her original outcome without any prompting from me, so I ask her:

And if *you had more energy,* **what would that be like?**
- It would mean having more economy in how I use it. Instead of frantically responding all the time (she mimes her version of overwhelm, turning rapidly from left to right and holding her head in her hands), I would be able to stay calm and focused (she faces straight ahead and does indeed look calm and focused, as if she's tapping back into that serenity she mentioned earlier).

She has intuitively made her own cognitive connection with the changes that have come largely unconsciously from the Clean Language and the bodywork. Staying calm and focused, a good kind of tiredness, peace and serenity and having more energy are all facets of the outcome that has emerged for her in this simple half-hour process. Before she goes, there's one more thing I want to remind her of.

And *the Rubik's cube,* **how is that now?**
- (Her eyes flick down, her head turns to the right. Another smile) I'm still sorting it out.

I move from Clean questions to asking her specifically about her hand movement:

Did you notice what your hands were doing when you mentioned it before?

Spontaneously she brings her hands back in front of her, one above the other, palms apart, fingers curved. I ask her what happens if she holds her hands like that and breathes down into the solar plexus area. As she tries it, I explain that this is a good way to recharge her batteries, to bring a bit of energy from every breath into the body's reservoirs where it can be stored for when it's needed. Perhaps I'm putting my own interpretation on her Rubik's cube; perhaps she'll forget all about this little exercise. But when a client's body seems to be signalling to me, using a vocabulary of movement that relates directly to her outcome, I think it's worth showing her what her bodymind seems to want her to know. I ask:

And how is that?
–   Calmer.

And when it's calmer, ***what happens*** to the Rubik's cube?
–   (She twists her wrists again very slightly and I see the hint of a smile) It's still sorting out, but it's as if the different parts of the cube are easier to move. They can slide around more easily.

And is that a good place to finish?
–   Yes.

That's one very simple example to get you thinking about how you might use Clean questions in your own kind of work. Of course, I didn't follow my eight steps exactly. How was I to know that she would start with her outcome ('To have more energy') and leave the problems (the tight neck, the tiredness and 'Frantically responding all the time') until we had almost finished? When you encourage people to open up to what's inside, things do get unpredictable, but in this case she used the first part of the session to connect with some very positive resources – the metaphor of the Rubik's cube, the whole new avenue opening up, the peace and serenity. This is a good example of one of the most important principles in Clean Language: as you guide your client through their internal landscape, the more you can help them connect with the positive resources they find there, and the easier it will be for them to work with the problems they want to resolve without experiencing the overwhelm those problems may be giving them in everyday life.

⁓ 21 ⁓

EXPLORING THE LANDSCAPE

The more Clean questions you ask, the more rich and detailed the client's awareness becomes of their own inner experience – a dynamic, internal reality with its own images, words, feelings and dimensions. Each question you ask leads your client further into this rarely visited internal landscape, and one of your jobs as the facilitator is to begin to map the territory and to keep track of the stages in the journey.

Say your client is a man who has come with a chronic pain in his knee joint. This is where your expedition begins. As you ask Clean questions, it can rapidly move on, for example, to a strange feeling in his lower back, and from there to a surprising sense of sadness which then becomes a metaphor – a cold fog that's hard to see through. When you ask if there's anything else about that cold fog that's hard to see through, he may say, 'No, it just stays there and it doesn't change.' At the same time, though, he becomes aware of a restricted feeling in his chest, which when you explore it, leads to deeper breathing and a pleasant but unfamiliar sensation of feeling of warmth there.

You ask, 'And that warmth inside the chest **is like what?**', and the client answers, 'Like little rays of sunshine'. Since you have been mapping the stages of the journey, you remember the fog, and realise that this might be a good place to ask the Relationship question – in this case, '**And is there a relationship between** little rays of sunshine coming from your heart **and** a cold fog that's hard to see through?'

You don't have to be a meteorologist to see how these two metaphors could indeed be related: that the sunshine – if it's strong enough – could dissipate the fog. In fact, as the practitioner, you might be tempted to try to make something happen by asking your client to imagine these little rays of sunshine beaming down on the cold fog. That might work and it might not, depending on the amount of energy, or neurological 'signal strength', the client is giving to the two different metaphors. If the little rays of sunshine are too weak to shift the cold fog, you could be setting him up to fail. It's also worth remembering that the fog might have qualities like softening something too harsh to see, or holding moisture that the dry earth needs, so trying to get rid of it may result in some kind of resistance.

Sometimes it's the client who tries to make something happen. Perhaps this man has done other kinds of visualisation work or is just very oriented to getting things done, and tries to get rid of something that arises in his internal landscape. You might ask, '**And is there anything else about** that cold fog?' He is silent for a while, then says, 'I've been imagining a wind that comes and blows it away.' This kind of active attempt to intervene in his own internal experience (to consciously conjure up a solution) may work temporarily but if it doesn't fit with the ecology of the rest of the client's symbolic landscape, then there will probably be some kind of mind/body message that tells him this – an intensifying of the original symptom or a new discomfort arising somewhere else in the body, or simply the stubborn refusal of the fog to be completely blown away. As the facilitator, it's your job to help the client notice these important but often subtle signals, to bring attention to them, amplifying the signal strongly enough for him to be able to recognise it as a genuine response from his own bodymind, something he can own, accept and work with.

Clean questions always come to your rescue when you need to do this. For example, you could ask:

And is there anything else about the stubborn refusal of the fog to be completely blown away?'
–   No, but the ache's come back in my lower back now.

And when the ache comes back in your lower back, *what happens to the fog?*
–   There are little patches of it still there, but when I go up to them, they move away, they keep their distance.

Distance always contains a hint of a relationship. Here your client has intuitively realised that there is some kind of negotiation going on with these stubborn patches of fog.

And when you stay a certain distance away, *then what happens?*
–   I see a kind of light inside.

And is there anything else about this light inside?
–   It has a warm glow – it's like there's this warm glow coming from the fog.

And what kind of warm glow is that?
–   It's like the difference between sunshine and moonlight. The fog is like moonlight and the glow is like sun shining through fog.

And what happens next?
–   Somehow this glow from the fog goes right into my chest.

And when it goes right into your chest, *then what happens?*
–   It's like the fog goes in with it, but it's okay. There's only a little bit of fog left, and the warm glow is going into my heart.

Your client is now fully engaged – almost as if he's watching a movie in his own private cinema. At moments like this, it's best just to remain silent or to keep things moving with utterly simple and reliable questions like '**And is there anything else…?**' or '**And what happens next?**'

And is there anything else about the fog going into your lungs, and the warm glow going into your heart?
- My heart gets warmer, and the fog goes into my lungs and keeps them cool.

You hear your client's voice slowing down and getting softer as he says this, and notice that he's breathing more deeply too. Another good moment to be invisibly present, remaining silent for a while before you ask:

And is there anything else about all that inside your chest?

He starts to smile gently and nods to himself, eyes closed, as if he's seeing the humour in some private joke.

- Not really, it just feels incredibly…

The words run out, the smile returns and you know the process has shifted to a different level. Usually you can feel it too, in yourself and in the space between you. You may be tempted to keep asking Clean questions but go very slowly and sensitively, since your client is probably moving into a more non-verbal kind of awareness. Another Clean question may help to amplify this even further, but since a question is by definition verbal, it may also distract him from where he needs to be right now. If you do ask another question, do it softly and slowly, so that his smile is there in the quality of your voice when you ask the next question. Alternatively, you can just say, 'And take the time you need just to stay with all of that…' This gives you some time to come back to yourself and leave your client in as Clean a space as possible.

As a mind/body therapist, once the process has got to this stage, what I'm really looking for is the point at which I can start working directly with the body and the energy channels in a way which will support the good changes which the Clean questions have begun. In this case the client has done a lot of work and made some powerful connections simply because the Clean questions have helped him focus his attention very precisely – first on different parts of his body, and then on different features of his inner landscape, and the relationships between them.

Meanwhile, part of your job is to think about how the client got to this place and where he started from. From the presenting knee problem, to the ache in the lower back, to the sadness, to the cold fog and the restricted breathing, to the feeling of warmth in the chest and the wordless smile: there are layers or stages in the journey of exploration that you have been on together. Whatever feelings, thoughts, memories or metaphors have emerged, they are all part of the client's inner landscape and need to be acknowledged and respected and held in awareness. An important part of your job as the facilitator is simply being able to retrace the steps of the journey in your head so that you can remind your client of how he got here, and encourage him to notice any relationships between these different parts of the landscape.

In the next chapter we'll look at how to do this, using Clean Language at the start to explore both problem and outcome, finding the point to transition into bodywork, and then coming back to Clean questions to help your client consolidate and clarify their whole experience, so that both verbal mind and bodymind have what they need.

22

TAKING LESS OF THE LOAD

A businessman in his late 50s has 'soft tissue damage' in his left ankle. At least, that's the label he has in his head, from what the physiotherapist told him. He is only in London for a few days but a mutual friend has suggested he come to see me. Six weeks before, he was piggybacking his granddaughter across the road when a sudden noise made him twist round. Instantly he felt his ankle give way and a lot of pain, but had to keep walking on it long enough to get her safely across the road. Although he's had three very effective acupuncture sessions, to stand or walk on it is still causing him pain.

I explain that before doing any bodywork it might be good, when something isn't healing up the way you'd expect it to, to find out if there is anything that still might need to be resolved. A few more questions reveal that he had a serious stroke a few years ago, after a prolonged divorce and in the middle of seeing through a major transformation in his business.

I ask him to settle down in his chair, to let his eyes relax and to take some time to notice the sensations of breathing, and then just to notice anything at all, any part of his body that might be drawing his attention.

– My shoulders – that's the first thing I notice; just a lot of tension there.

We explore that tension a little more; where exactly it is, what kind of tension. When I ask if there's anything else about that tension in the shoulders, something interesting happens.

– There's something there in my ankle now.

And were you aware of that before?
– No.

And what kind of something is that in your ankle?
– It feels tight.

And is there anything else about tight?
– There's a red colour to it.

And when it feels tight and there's a red colour to it, is there anything else?
– There's a tingling.

What kind of tingling?
– There's a sort of vibration there, a pulsing.

And where is that vibration, that pulsing?
– On the inner side; it feels like heat.

And when there's vibration, and pulsing, and it feels like heat on the inner side of your ankle, then what happens?
– It's probably about protecting it.

Suddenly we have moved from physical sensations to an interpretation, but the word 'probably' makes me wonder if the idea is a real communication from the body or if it's the client making a deliberate effort to come up with an explanation. Sometimes clients do this when they're not sure what the Clean questions are all about and they want to please the practitioner. I'm sure that's not the case here, but a good question to ask is:

And what tells you that?
- There's some tension in my shoulders.

What kind of tension?
- It feels like it's protecting me. ·

And what kind of protecting?
- It doesn't want me to do it again.

Maybe the 'it' refers to piggybacking his granddaughter across a busy road, or maybe it refers to something else, but I don't need to know. All I need to do is ask:

And is there anything else about that 'it' that the protecting doesn't want you to do again?

He is silent for a while. There is a sigh and a very slight shudder through the whole left side of his body. Then he answers the question:

- I thought it was just about what happened, twisting round like that with my granddaughter on my back.

He's silent. I'm silent. I can't think of a question to ask, and I don't think I need to. He's just taking his time.

- I can feel this little throbbing in the side of my head. I have that sometimes since the stroke.

And is there anything else about that little throbbing?
- Actually it's about taking less of the load.

Taking less of the load?
- Uh-huh.

And can you take less of the load?
- I don't know.

Can you imagine taking less of the load?
- Maybe.

And then what happens?
- (He sighs again) It's kind of releasing something around here (he puts a hand on his diaphragm area).

And is there anything else about releasing something around there?

The only answer he gives is a soft, 'Uh-huh'. His lips part slightly and he seems to be drifting into semi-consciousness. Then after a few gentle snores, he is back. So I ask:

And what just happened?
- I don't know.

And how is it where your hand is now (around his diaphragm)?
- Good. It feels good.

And is there a relationship between releasing something around there **and** taking less of the load?

He is silent again. A colder silence. Have I asked one question too many? His jaw tightens and his eyes close again. I come back to my own breathing and get a sense of a clear boundary all round him. When I connect with it, it seems to say, 'Back off'. Maybe this has something to do with the protection he's talking about. After a long time, he says:

- Can you ask me that again?

And is there a relationship between releasing something around there **and** taking less of the load?
- Yeah, maybe there is.

His eyes moisten and there's emotion in his voice, but it still feels like there's a boundary here that he would prefer me not to cross. Or is this issue of taking less of the load the real reason for his visit? I don't know, but if I stay Clean, I can leave the choice to him.

And when you just imagine taking less of the load, *then what happens?*
- The tension in my right shoulder is going.

And just staying with that sense of the tension in your right shoulder going...*then what happens?*
- Then it starts relaxing in my left shoulder too.

We're back on terra firma, back where we began with the tension in his shoulders. The physical sensations are responding and I feel the protective boundary disappearing. Now it's time to check if there's a relationship between the shoulders and the original symptom.

And when your left shoulder relaxes, *what happens* in your left ankle?
- The pain's reduced there quite a lot. It feels lighter.

Anything else about lighter?
- It's not a knotted-up mess.

And when it's not a knotted-up mess, *then what happens?*
- It's a different colour...like yellow. It certainly isn't red.

And when it's like yellow, *what happens?*
- My left thigh feels tight.

And where is that tight in your left thigh coming from?
- Do you mean philosophically or physically?

I meant physically, but when the client introduces another possibility, always give them the option of exploring it.

Whichever makes sense to you.
- It's providing strength for my ankle.

What kind of strength?
- My whole left leg is tingling now.

He smiles and shakes his head gently as if bemused by the way his body is responding. He's silent for quite a while as he stays with the tingling. My sense as I watch is that the protective energy is really releasing. His shoulders are gently widening out, and something seems to be relaxing in his left hip. All this, of course, without any actual bodywork from me yet.

- The pain level in my ankle is a lot less now than when we started.

Would that be a good place for you to lie down?
- Yes. If I can get the rest of my body to relax like that, it would be exactly what I need.

In the treatment, he is at first quite alert to the different sensations his body is giving him as I work various points. Whatever it means to him to take less of the load, he is really noticing how much tension his body has been holding onto, not just in his shoulders but in his lower back too. Then he drifts off again into the semi-asleep state he was briefly in before, his jaw softening and his breathing becoming slower and deeper.

As we near the end of the session, I think back through all the steps of the process we have just been through: the way his ankle responded to the first Clean questions, the tightness, the red colour, the tingling, the pulsing and the sense of heat on the inner side; then his sense that it had to do with protection, which was connected to the tension in his shoulders, and then taking less of the load, the question about whether that was possible, his attention being drawn to the diaphragm, and the emotion that he felt. He seemed to have taken some decision silently, which allowed all that protective tension to release.

So what do I still need to ask? According to my 8-step process, I'm at step 5. What I need to do now is ask him how he is and remind him of his original outcome. Only now I realise that I never actually asked the Outcome question. His body seemed to be answering it for him, step by step, until he arrived at that outcome of taking less of the load.

I ask him how he is now and he says that he can't feel any pain in his ankle. When he stands up and takes a few steps, he says it feels like a real improvement.

And *taking less of the load?*
- (He smiles) Yeah, I'm on it.

I'm not sure what he means by that, but I think he is.

And is that a good place to finish?
- Yeah, thanks. I'll let you know how it goes.

The next day he emails to say: 'Thanks for the session…my ankle is 200 per cent better.'

Four days later, back home by then, he emails again, 'I just wanted to say my ankle is 100 per cent better.' I'm not quite sure of the mathematics, but it sounds like it worked. We all have sessions like this sometimes, when the client arrives in serious pain and leaves with much less or none at all. And of course it can happen without using any Clean Language at all. But I think this case is a good example of three ways that Clean questions can help: first, it shows how much of the work the client can do before the actual bodywork begins; second, it shows how useful the questions can be in helping the client explore any underlying issues; and finally, it shows how Clean Language, carefully used, can help us to respect our client's privacy around those issues, while still being a very effective aid to resolving them.

3.2 A CLEAN APPROACH TO TRAUMA

In London, where I live, it still sometimes happens that builders excavating the foundations of a site uncover an unexploded wartime bomb. The same can happen in a bodywork session. Suddenly the client's breathing stops, their muscles tense and their eyes spring open as the vagus system is either hijacked by the sympathetic nervous system into fight/flight, or switched from its restorative role into the freeze/faint response. When it does, we need to remember the skills of the bomb disposal expert – sensitivity, steadiness of nerve and an instant readiness to back off gently at the slightest sign of danger. This applies all the more when you use Clean Language, since just three or four questions can uncover long buried and potentially explosive things. At the same time, we need to remember that working with trauma was originally what prompted David Grove to develop Clean Language. Realising that many clients found it easier to work with a trauma metaphorically than by going directly back into the memory itself, he crafted his original list of Clean questions to help them explore their own metaphorical landscape with as little interference as possible from the therapist. Through metaphor, he helped trauma victims recover their lives because he knew that sometimes metaphors can be literally life-saving.

I realised this when I saw a TV documentary in which a naval bomb disposal officer described what happened when an enemy missile tore through the hull of his ship and penetrated deep into its hold without actually exploding. Examining it, he gradually realised that the only way he could neutralise it would be to lift it up and carry it to the deck, where it could be carefully lowered into the sea. As his fingers began to feel for the steadiest way to hold it, he found himself imagining that the bomb was a sleeping baby and that all he had to do was to carry it gently enough, one step at a time, to get it on deck without waking it up. Wherever that metaphor came from, it probably saved his life and the lives of many others. When a trauma arises as I work with a client, that image sometimes comes back to me. Trauma can indeed have a ferocious explosive power, but at the same time, we need the tenderness of hand and steadiness of heart to be able to cradle it like a sleeping child before we can get it to a place where it is safe to work with.

Fortunately, over the past 30 years, trauma pioneers like Bessel van der Kolk (2014), Peter Levine (1997, 2010), Pat Ogden (Ogden and Fisher 2015) and Babette Rothschild (2000) have created safe and reliable procedures for treating clients and training practitioners, and at the same time our notion of trauma has evolved considerably. From something that was once thought of as only happening to victims of extreme violence or abuse, it is probably accepted now by most therapists that we are all full of mini-traumas – 'the thousand natural shocks that flesh is heir to' (as Hamlet put it) – and that they are a natural hazard of being human, something we have all experienced to some degree and which we adapt to, ignore or cope with as best we can. Then, when something happens that reminds us of a trauma still held somewhere inside us, Clean Language can help us find the metaphor that can safely defuse its explosive potential. In the next four case studies, we look at some of the ways that traumatic memories can re-surface unexpectedly in a bodywork session and how Clean Language can help clients to integrate those memories when they do.

23

THE TIDAL WAVE OF TRAUMA

It often happens that an old trauma surfaces in relation to some setback a client has experienced recently in their everyday life. The purpose here is to show how Clean questions can help both client and practitioner get clearer about the often complex web of connections that the mind and memory can weave between a childhood trauma and adult experience.

My client is a man in his mid-30s who has recently achieved great success in his career after several intensely demanding years' working on a particular project. But the pressure took its toll. Six months ago he began to experience memory loss and intense anxiety. He had a brain scan but the doctors were unable to diagnose or offer any treatment. We have been doing regular sessions over the past two months and, to my surprise, these symptoms have almost completely disappeared. He is back at work full-time on a demanding new project. His main concern in this session, he says, is how bad he's been feeling after a meeting with his boss, in which he felt he was being 'told off' and was accused of behaving childishly and 'like a victim' in a disagreement about how to solve a particular production problem with another member of the team.

Thinking about it, he says, made him realise, 'I've always been in front of the headmaster, being misunderstood and always thinking that I'm right.' He's also had some unusual lower back pain this week. When I ask him what he would like to have happen, he says, 'I want to find out what kind of person I really am.'

As he's talking, my attention is drawn to a sense of something fragile and wobbly around his pelvis, while his upper body seems hefty and a little hunched. I ask:

Is there anything else about *finding out what kind of person I really am?*

As so often happens, his next answer shifts from talking about what he does want, to what he doesn't want.

- I don't want to argue with so many people – my boss, my partner, my dad…

He pauses for a moment, seeing a pattern, and then says:

- …men who are important, or important to me.

And what would that be like, *if you didn't argue with so many men who are important to you?*
- (He leans back in his chair, suddenly looking much more relaxed) It would be more fun, and less aggressive.

And is there anything else about *more fun and less aggressive?*
- I'm aware of my shoulders being hunched – that you get into a victim posture when you think you need to be aggressive. So he's right, in a way, my boss.

As he says this, he deliberately shifts into an exaggeratedly hunched posture, defensive and yet looking as if he's ready to lash out.

I ask if there's anything else about the victim posture. He looks down and is silent for a long time, beginning to focus more on his breathing and his body – a mindfulness exercise we did in a previous session. In the silence, I can see his shoulders softening, and energy moving down through his body. The fragile look I noticed before seems now to be centred in his lower back. We have already explored things enough with Clean questions to have set some real changes in motion, so I ask if this would be a good point for him to lie down, and he agrees.

As he gets himself comfortable, lying on his back, I switch out of Clean mode and into mindfulness mode, talking a little about the breath being an anchor which is always there to bring us back to the body. Picking up on the metaphor, he says:

- When these emotions come, it's difficult not to be swept away by the huge wave.

He's silent again for a few breaths, eyes closed. I'm struck by the image, because it corresponds so well with what I'm feeling as I explore that fragile feeling in his lower back. According to the Chinese Five Elements system, we've both been using metaphors about Water. Physically, this element relates to the spine and the lower back; the emotion it relates to is fear. As I press my hand into his lower back, he's surprised at how tender it is there.

Working on the lumbar area leads me up to the neck, where something is holding on in a way that won't respond to anything my hands can offer. For me, this is always a sign that I need to hand the initiative back to the client, to ask another question rather than trying to solve the problem myself. Meanwhile, he says he's feeling his lower back get more and more painful. There is an edge of fear in his voice. Have my fingers released too much down there? I take a breath, re-ground myself and ask him where exactly it feels more painful. This one Clean question is all he needs to remember the trauma, and the fear disappears from his voice as he tells the story:

- My parents sent me to boarding school when I was eight years old. It was a progressive type of school and they were very into all that. I went off one day on my own to explore a beach that we'd been told we should never go to on our own because it wasn't safe. I didn't understand about tides, and realised too late that I was on a bit of sand that the water had already cut off from the shore. I thought if I stayed there and shouted loud enough and long enough, someone might hear me, but then I thought that if they found me then I would get into trouble for being on the beach in the first place. So I started wading back through the water. I was determined to get back on my own, without anyone finding out, but I didn't realise how strong the current was. I was probably only in the water less than ten minutes, but it got deeper and deeper, and colder and colder, and I was absolutely terrified. I couldn't see the bottom and once I nearly went under and I remember this feeling like I was totally insignificant and the water really didn't care whether I lived or died. When I got to the shore, I literally collapsed. It must have been the cold and the shock combined.

When I woke up again, I lay there for a while wondering if I was still alive. I was terribly scared. Eventually I managed to stand up. I could walk but only very slowly, and when I finally got back to the school, I couldn't tell anyone about it because the head had told us not to go there in the first place.

As he tells the story, I'm working deep into his lower back muscles, trying to be as Clean with my touch as I am with the language. My fingers do a kind of deep listening that seems to work better than any kind of active treatment to make it feel safe enough for muscles and body tissues to release embedded trauma. The sequence of feelings my fingers pick up is first a kind of unresponsive stiffness, at its worst an almost dead feeling; then a sense of something very slightly opening and softening; then a hint of movement, of energy flowing back into the channels – my fingertips changing their positions, sometimes by just a millimetre, to be exactly where they need to be – and then a feeling of life returning, of the muscles regaining tone and elasticity and feeling again like they're part of the rest of the body rather than islands of resistance within it.

Then I return to the stuck feeling in his neck. This time it's ready to release the shock that still seems to be echoing in the bones at the back of his skull.

As I finish the bodywork, I ask how he is. He says it felt like 'a tidal wave of mortal fear' releasing. It seems that what we both realise as we talk about it is how closely the traumatic memory mirrors his current problem – his childlike desire to explore the world in his own way (one of the things that people most admire about his professional work) and his sense of some unfathomable vulnerability when confronting male authority figures. His body was not just remembering the physical trauma but was associating it with what happens when that authority is defied.

When I ask him to come back to the problem with his boss – he had a meeting scheduled with him the following week – he realises that now he feels quite matter-of-fact about it. He can't see a problem in putting his professional point of view, and fighting for it, and he is ready to acknowledge that he used over-emotive language and to apologise for that.

When he came for his next session two weeks later, I checked with him about the meeting and he said it had been fine, 'All very grown up'. But he'd been in bed for two days after the last session, 'completely run down, exhausted, in bed sweating as if I had flu, but I didn't. It was like all that stuff from the session working its way through.' And his lower back? He had been very aware of it when he was ill, he said, but funnily enough, after the meeting with his boss he'd stopped noticing it and he hadn't felt any pain there since.

That pain in his back returned a few times in the year that followed, but not as severely as before, and he learned to respond to it as a warning sign that the tidal waters of his very demanding working life might be threatening to cut him off again. And over that same year I noticed, and so did he, that when he talked about getting into arguments with important men in his life, he no longer allowed his anger to sweep him away.

~ 24 ~

ANGRY RED BLOTCHES

This next example of how Clean questions can help in working with trauma comes from a very experienced colleague who uses Clean Language together with a number of bodywork therapies that she has integrated over the years. Here she tells in her own words how Clean questions helped her to get to the core of her client's bewildering array of symptoms.

My client is a woman in her early 60s who suffers from chest pains, digestive problems, pain in her knee joints, occasional severe headaches, and anger with her mother, 'For dying young and not being there to protect me from sexual abuse I suffered a few years later'.

Various medical tests have been all clear, and she says she has done some psychotherapy which helped her a lot. Her long list of symptoms gives me some obvious diagnostic clues, but at the same time, with so many symptoms, I'm wondering where to start and how I can really help. When I ask what she would like to have happen she says, 'Oh yes, and there is this other thing. Every time I take my six-year-old granddaughter to the park, I get these angry red blotches come up on my skin and I get desperate to get home again. Once I'm back indoors I have to wash my face with soap and water just to calm them down again. Nobody else knows about it except my granddaughter, and she just laughs when she sees them, and calls me 'Spotty'. I deliberately drive her to parks that are miles away, so I won't meet anyone I know. My daughter thinks I'm a bit odd doing that, but I haven't told her why, and I haven't told the doctor either because I don't want her thinking I'm OCD. It's just so embarrassing.'

The more I ask her about these angry red blotches and listen to her describing in detail what happens, the more I feel at a loss to make any real sense of it. I would feel like a complete fraud saying, 'Just lie yourself down, and I'm sure we'll have that cleared up in no time.' So I ask her:

And what happens just before *you get those angry red blotches?*
– I get this complete panic.

And where is *that panic?*
– I've no idea. It just comes.

Where *do you feel it?*

She goes very quiet for a while and when I ask what's happening, she says she can see herself as a child.

What's she like?
– She's feeling filthy.

How old is she?
– Six.

And what does *that six-year-old who's feeling filthy* *want to have* *happen?*
– To get out of the park.

And is there anything else about *get out of the park?*

Tears stream down her face as she explains. She had worked on the abuse in her psychotherapy and thought that it was 'Done and dusted' and that the only issue now was her anger with her mother, which she couldn't do anything about since she couldn't blame her mother for things that had happened after her death. But what she is realising now is that the abuse happened in a park, the same park that she'd always loved to go to with her mother when she was alive. Apparently she had made no connection before between the abuse and her panic at being in a park and getting the angry red blotches.

*And when you know that now, **what would you like to have happen?***
- (She sits up straighter for a moment staring straight ahead) To be able to take my granddaughter to the park without feeling terrified.

After the bodywork part of the session, I ask, 'So how do you feel now?' She says she feels a lot more relaxed. I ask what happens when she thinks about going to the park. To my surprise, she laughs, a girlish, giggly laugh. 'I don't know about that,' she says, 'but I'm not expecting any miracles!'

I wasn't expecting any miracles either, and in the next two more sessions she didn't seem to want to talk much, so I kept the Clean Language to a minimum, focusing on the bodywork because that seemed to be what she wanted. I did check with her about going to the park, but she said she hadn't had to look after her granddaughter lately because they were away on holiday.

Then, to my surprise, the day after the third session, she emailed to say that she'd decided to do 'a test run' and had gone to the park by herself. She couldn't believe that she'd felt no panic at all, and no angry red blotches. In the following weeks, the blotches came back when she took her granddaughter to the park, but she said they were less 'angry'. I asked if there was a relationship between 'less angry' and how she felt towards her mother, and she realised that the red blotches were now more to do with her anxiety about protecting her six-year-old granddaughter. As we carried on with our sessions, the blotches eventually disappeared completely.

What was so valuable about using Clean Language in that first session was that it gave me the clarity of intention I needed to feel confident that the bodywork would help, possibly saving months of puzzlement and confusion for us both.

~ 25 ~

I WILL DIE TOO

Trauma is not just about horrific events. It can also be caused by apparently innocent remarks, as in this example when a mother has simply tried to give an honest answer to her daughter's question. In this case, my client already knows Clean Language – she has studied it to help her in her work as a business coach – and she uses my Clean questions the way an energetic hiker uses a walking stick – each question giving her a little extra push to help her on her way. At first it seems like her problem is one we can all experience working with clients, and that we probably all have our sticking-plaster remedies for. But with the help of Clean questions she is able to move beyond that kind of remedy-seeking into far more subjective territory, taking herself back to a very personal memory and to the resources she needs to resolve it.

I ask her where she would like to begin. Her cheerful expression immediately turns into a frown.

– I get angry with my clients.

As she says this, she touches the space between her eyebrows. Of course, in some healing traditions this is a very significant spot – the 'third eye' – but it may also simply be that she feels some tension there. It is not my job at this point to make any judgements about the gesture, but it's very important to note it since every unconscious gesture, including ones made right at the start of a session, may be attempts by the bodymind to communicate directly with you, the practitioner.

- On one hand (she says) I want to be caring and to understand them from the heart, but on the other hand if they keep coming back complaining about the same issue over and over, I want to say 'So what are you going to do about it?' And I get angry (here both her hands come together as fists) and then the client gets angry.

How often does this happen?
- It happens with every client at some point.

I ask her to give me some examples, and she mentions three clients and how she has got angry with each of them at some point.

- I feel guilty about it.

And when** you get angry with every client at some point, and you feel guilty about it, **what would you like to have happen?
- (She gestures to her chest) It gets very tight here, as if it's saying, 'You have to be more compassionate.' Then I feel pressure in my chest.

And then what happens?
- I don't breathe properly.

***And is there anything else** when you don't breathe properly?*
- There's a burden on my upper back.

And then what happens?
- It feels tight in my hips and pelvis.

What kind of tight?
- There's a pressure in my solar plexus like a ball going around and around inside.

And when all of that, **what would you like to have happen?**

She gives herself time to let her body respond to the question, noticing each shift as it comes.

- My spine aligned, feet on the ground, shoulders open. Breathing.

And when all of that, **then what happens?**
- Now it's here (she gestures to her throat).

And what's there?
- There's tightness.

What kind of tightness?
- As if there's an obstacle there, as if my throat's not connected to my chest.

This is the first point at which I might think, 'Ah, there's an obstacle, a block, something not connecting. This might be a good place to start some bodywork.' But let's remember that Clean questions are themselves a form of bodywork, and see what happens if I ask one more. Since there is a problem, some version of the Outcome question seems appropriate:

And when your throat's not connected to your chest, **what needs to happen?**
- To feel lighter in my throat, more spacious.

She keeps her right hand on her chest as she explores this further.

- On the left side of my throat it feels like there's dust.

What kind of dust?
- It's yellow and heavy.

She coughs loudly, as if she really does have something in her throat.

–   Now I have the same feeling down here, dusty and yellow.

She gestures to her lower left abdomen, and coughs again.

Coughs are rarely accidental once a Clean session has begun, and it's important to include any sound your client makes into your next question. So I ask:

And when it's dusty and yellow down there, and that cough, **what happens next?**
–   It's telling me that everything is going to be alright and it's here to remind me of something.

What kind of something?
–   I don't know but it feels very good in my chest now – as if it has space and can express what it needs to express.

And your throat now?
–   It's things I haven't said; the things I've swallowed.

What kind of things?
–   The need to be liked and to say yes.

And in your lower abdomen?
–   Ha! It says, 'Whatever you swallow is stored there.'

And then what happens?
–   It's like something that doesn't belong here.

And what kind of something doesn't belong here?
–   It doesn't belong to me.

And when it doesn't belong to you, **what needs to happen?**
–   I can express my opinion without the fear of rejection and without fear the other person will be hurt.

And then what happens?
–   I feel a release going right up through my body.

Anything else about that release?
- It has a voice. The voice says, 'Come together and we'll see what's going on'.

She seems to have arrived at a natural resting place. Without any further question from me, she takes a minute to check how she is.

- I feel safe in my chest…and my throat is connected to the rest of my body…my mind is more relaxed…and my neck is more relaxed too. It feels flowing and smooth on both sides of my neck.

She pauses now, eyes closed, still paying close attention to what is going on inside. No need to interrupt; if I did, it would only be to satisfy my own curiosity. Eventually she speaks:

- I can feel this flow going right down to my feet.

She has already made so many changes, mentally as well as bodily, it's as if she has already had a treatment. This seems like a good moment to come back to her original issue of getting angry with her clients. I ask her again about each of the three clients who she mentioned earlier. When she thinks about them now, she acts out something different for each one, getting insights into what each one really needs for their own anger to be acknowledged.

I ask if this would be a good point to start the shiatsu treatment, and she agrees.

And if there was a place you would like some kind of contact, where would that be?
- Here in my abdomen.

I put my hand there. It feels agitated and confused. So I silently ask myself a Clean question, '**And when** it's agitated and confused, **that's like what?**' The answer comes back as an image in my mind's eye; something dark and spiralling – a kind of vortex, perhaps even a tornado.

Meanwhile, as she focuses her attention there, she says that it's moved to her head. She has a headache.

The more she listens to her body, the more it seems to know exactly what it wants to do next, so I adjust my Clean questions accordingly.

And would *your head* **like some kind of touch?**
- I can't think – it makes my headache worse.

She pauses, eyes closed, just breathing.

- Very hot in my forehead. It's like a hammer on the upper part of my head.

Something strong is happening here, but there seems to be no desire from her head for any direct help from me. My hand is still on her abdomen, feeling changes there. All I need to do is check whether this is part of a pattern she already knows.

And is that a familiar feeling?
- Yes, when I'm very tired.

As she focuses on it, it moves down to her lower abdomen again. She breathes down into it a few times, then says, 'It's like a storm passing.'

What kind of *storm?*
- I need protection.

What kind of *protection?*

Suddenly she is in tears, a real raw burst of fierce emotion. There is no point asking her anything while this is going on, so I just stay as present as I can, while the storm passes.

- I don't get migraines much any more, but I started to get them after a conversation with my mother when I was six years old. I was asking her about death and why people die. She said that everyone dies in the end, and I asked, 'What about you?' She said, 'One day, I will die too.' Now I feel like that six-year-old me again.

And what does that six-year-old you feel?
- Scared to death and cut off at the knees. I've lost that grounded feeling.

Her tears come again, even more fierce than before. After a while, I ask:

And with all of this, what would you like to have happen?

As she thinks about how to answer, she notices something is already happening.

- I feel something like surgery is going on in my knees. I had knee pain for many years; it was always connected with my period.

Anything else about that connection with your period?
- The loss of blood.

Anything else about that loss of blood?
- Like something being lost, and fear of loss. Only now am I making that connection.

And what happens when you do?
- I feel the sacrum is very hot.

Spontaneously she turns onto her side, as if she knows her body needs to be in that position. After a while, she says:

- I feel a connection from the sacrum to the third eye.

Remember: this is the first place she touched when she mentioned her original problem; a real confirmation that the first gesture your client makes in a session can often be a clue about everything else that is going to happen. And now she is aware of it and names it:

- It's like the third-eye space has been cleared. The heat in the sacrum feels okay – it goes into the belly and internal organs.

And then what happens?
- My mother didn't express feelings with hugs and kisses. I missed that as a child. I needed more hugs – to be touched by her.

A little bit of history, a piece of a narrative, has suddenly found its way into the dialogue. It sounds well-rehearsed, a familiar thought. I search for a simple question which will help her connect this old sense of self with all the changes she has just been making.

And if you'd had more hugs?
- I'd feel self-confident without struggling.

She stays with that for a moment. All this time I have been making gentle connections with my hands to each part of her body that seemed to be asking to be touched, but now my hand has come back to her abdomen. The tornado-like vortex that was there before has settled down, and under my palm it feels peaceful now. As I stay with that connection, she says:

- I did seven years of psychotherapy and this is what I was looking for – reassuring touch, without so much talking.

And when you have reassuring touch without so much talking, then what happens?
- I feel good.

And where do you feel good?
- In my lower abdomen – it feels like it's sufficient.

When something has changed for the better, and the client is aware of that, it's time to reconnect with the original problem.

And when it feels sufficient there, what is that like for the six-year-old you?
- I will die too.

She says this in a gentle tone, not a despairing one. There's a simple sense of acceptance in it so I ask the obvious question:

And then what happens, when you will die too?
- We will meet again.

And when you meet again?
- We will hug.

Tears come again, but these are very different tears. The storm is long passed. They just quietly roll down her cheeks, and I feel my own heart softening and opening with the pure energy of this reunion.

We talk a bit after the treatment about all that has come up for her. She says she feels now that her anger with her clients was like an alarm, like her six-year-old self wanting to say to her mother, 'What are you going to do in order not to die?'

We need to check what's different now in her relationship with the original problem.

And what would you do now when you start feeling angry with a client?
–   I would ask them what they would like to have happen.

She gestures with open palms. I mirror the gesture and ask if there's anything else about those open palms.

–   Respect. And something deep that comes from here (gesturing to her lower abdomen).

What kind of something?
–   There is a sense of relief there.

And there? (I gesture towards her third eye.)
–   I will see them as they really are.

She pauses, imagining that and looking straight ahead. Then she rubs her knees (those knees that felt like they'd had some kind of surgery), smiles and says:

–   A long journey!

And would that be a good place to finish?
–   Yes!

She came back to see me a couple of months later and I asked how things had been since our last session. The first thing she said was that she was much more aware of the power of hugging:

- Yesterday my three-year-old nephew was kicking me as I put on his clothes. Instinctively, I put him on my lap and hugged him and he stopped kicking. Then I remembered what happened in my session with you and it was crystal clear to me that hugging is so precious for children, and how much it helps them develop self-confidence, and how it nourishes us as adults. So I've been embracing him a lot more and feeling a warm light between us.

When I asked how things had been with her clients, she said she'd realised that the anger was not just hers but theirs too; that her frustration at them not changing was a reflection of their own frustration at not being able to change.

- For example, with one client, I realised that the pressure the company was putting on me to get results with him was part of my frustration too. Frustration with myself. So you could say, I was able to make a Cleaner space for him. After that he was able to do the same, to listen to his anger. We worked on that and it made a real difference, for him and for everyone in his team.

~ 26 ~

DROPPING THE BABY

Any kind of technique, including Clean Language, which aims to treat trauma by bringing attention to the symptoms of trauma, runs the risk of amplifying those symptoms. Traumatic incidents often strengthen negative beliefs that were already there before the event, anchoring themselves more deeply in the bodymind. It's also very natural to develop anxiety about when those symptoms of trauma might return, in the same way that a depressive episode can be triggered simply by worrying about the possibility of having one.

This case study shows how one traumatic event can affect a person at several different levels. This client has a history of panic attacks, which we have been working on for more than a year. Now the attacks are far less frequent and less intense, and she has much more confidence in her ability to recognise and manage the symptoms as soon as they begin. But there's been a five-month gap in our sessions after she gave birth to her first baby, and she's been experiencing severe anxiety without knowing where it's coming from.

As we work she remembers the traumatic event and discovers not only a belief that it was bound to happen but also a fear that it could happen again; meanwhile a voice inside her tells her to stay permanently on guard and not give in to the emotions that are still there from the trauma itself.

During the session, her body is registering these different beliefs and emotions literally at different levels, from her throat to her lower abdomen. Using a combination of Clean Language and shiatsu, we follow the trail her bodymind seems to be offering us, connecting felt sensations with beliefs and emotions, and allowing some deep healing to occur.

She arrives and talks first about life with her baby. Things are going well, but in the last couple of weeks she has been experiencing severe anxiety. When she made the appointment with me a few days ago, she says, her anxiety level was 'through the roof' but it's calmed down a bit now. When I ask her to rate it from one to ten, she says that for the past couple of days it's been about seven. Interestingly, she mentions that she had a really strong massage recently that had made the anxiety much worse without bringing any improvement later.

'How much worse?' I ask, and she says that afterwards she felt a total disconnection from her body, and that for a day or two she needed to hold onto something to contain the anxiety; it was hard to breathe, and even hard to swallow food. Her explanation for all this anxiety, and for her negative reaction to the massage, is her past history of anxiety combining with all the pressures of being a new mother. 'I've been sleep-deprived for weeks and running on adrenaline,' she says, throwing her arms up and her head back and widening her eyes in imitation of a classic startle response.

I ask if she'd like to lie down and explore this anxiety a bit further to see if her body has any clues about where it might be coming from. She is happy to do that and when she's comfortable and as relaxed as the anxiety allows, I ask:

And with all of this, what are are you drawn to most?
- I've got a bit of low-level anxiety in my tummy.

And is there anything else about that low-level anxiety?
- It's like butterflies, and my throat feels tight.

And which of those draws you most, the butterflies or the throat?
- My throat.

And what happens next in your throat?

After a long pause, she says:

- It's releasing.

And when it's releasing in the throat, *what happens to* the butterflies?

After a few seconds, she lets out a big breath.

And what happened just before that breath?
- I just realised I *could* stay with the butterflies. I didn't want to, but when you said that, I did.

And when you can stay with the butterflies, *then what happens?*

She is silent again, eyes closed as she really focuses on what's happening in her body.

- The butterflies go away, then they pop back as soon as I think they're gone.

There is something unusual about these butterflies, I think. They're not behaving like her normal anxiety symptoms do. Those tend to get more intense as soon as she focuses on them, and then gradually fade away. These butterflies seem to be playing hide and seek; they keep coming back once she's forgotten about them.

Are they there now?
- Yes.

Slipping out of Clean Language and into a more deliberately therapeutic kind of question, I ask:

And is it okay just to breathe down into where they are, and let them know you're paying attention to them, and to see how they respond?

After only a few seconds, she suddenly says:

– Ah! A little trip to A&E is coming back to me.

She has suddenly remembered that about three months ago, when the baby was just eight weeks old, her husband was carrying him upstairs and slipped; the baby fell onto the hard wood floor.

'For ten seconds, I thought he was dead,' she says, and the weight of those ten seconds is suddenly very present in the room. Then she fills in the silence with what was going through her head in those moments. 'When it happened, it was as if I'd been waiting for it to happen,' she says, 'as if it's all too good to be true, and you're wondering when the bad thing's going to happen.'

Now, she says, she feels anxiety every time her husband carries the baby upstairs.

And where is that anxiety?
– In my chest.

And is it there now?

She's silent for a couple of breaths, checking.

– It feels okay.

And when it feels okay, is there anything else about that anxiety in the chest?
– What I'd really like is to cry, but I can't.

At this point I get my first signal from her bodymind that it wants me to start work, and the point calling me to touch it is on the upper spine. Two points actually, on the channel of energy that runs right up the centre of the spine, and as I hold them I ask her to keep her attention on that feeling in her chest that she'd like to cry but can't. At first, these two points, which have a close connection with the heart, feel tight and protective. After a while though, they relax and to my surprise begin to feel soft and open. I ask her, **'What just happened?'** She says she suddenly started seeing an image of her baby's smiling face, and thinking how loveable he is.

And when you see his smiling face and think how loveable he is, **what happens** *in your chest?*
– It's fine there now. The anxiety's moved down to here.

She gestures to her upper abdomen. I move my hand there, feeling another kind of tightness. Time for another Clean question.

And where does this anxiety **come from?**
– From the fear that it might happen again.

And is there anything else about that fear?
– It's like being on your guard. Like there's no time for self-indulgent things like crying.

Sometimes all it takes is just to listen to yourself; to hear yourself find the words that describe some vague but persistent sensation. This seems to be one way that the verbal mind can be invaluable in healing. It seems that to give a name to what was previously only felt has allowed something to be released. This time, I feel the tightness begin to soften in her upper abdomen just before she says it. Then, as she processes the idea that 'there's no time for self-indulgent things like crying,' she notices her upper abdomen begins to feel okay and the feeling is now moving right down to her lower belly. My fingers find the point that feels most empty, a deep kind of emptiness, the sort that comes from running on adrenaline with a new baby and having acute anxiety attacks at the same time, and believing that you must always be on guard and that there's no time for self-indulgent things like crying. My hand stays on this point for a long time, until gradually it begins to fill up again, like a dry well filling with fresh water.

Meanwhile, she has drifted off into a gentle sleep. That stern protector, the part of her that thinks she should always be on guard, seems to have decided that just for the moment it's okay to relax. I carry on working and after about ten minutes, she wakes up again, saying she feels like she's just had a week of rest.

After the treatment, I ask her about how she is now in relation to the anxiety. She says that it feels okay, about a three out of ten, but adds, 'There will always be a bit of it still there.'

When I see her again a month later, she says the anxiety continued for a couple of days after the last session, 'But I decided not to panic and to trust that the treatment would work, and after a few days, it did. Since then it's been much better.'

I ask myself whether the treatment had any real effect, since it was only when she decided to trust that it *would* work that things began to change. But there is usually a logic to the way the bodymind tries to resolve things. It may not be the same kind of logic that the verbal mind would recognise, but it makes its own kind of sense.

In the first session, after remembering how her husband dropped the baby, she intuitively came up with a powerful way of resourcing herself. When she imagined the smiling face of her baby in her mind's eye, and thought how loveable he was, she no longer had the feeling of wanting to cry.

In her next session, she felt a lot of tension in the diaphragm area, around her solar plexus. Something inside me responded to that; I started feeling very grounded and very still, and the story of the bomb disposal expert (see page 209) popped into my head. As I held my hand just above her solar plexus, she suddenly felt an involuntary spasm ripple through the muscles there. A few more followed, but with no emotions, as if something was being released at a very physical level. After that session, her anxiety calmed down considerably, and on the one occasion that it reappeared in the following month, in a crowded restaurant with friends, she was able to deal with it easily by stepping outside to breathe fresh air.

From my point of view, perhaps the most important thing she took from that first session was the sense that she could actively decide what attitude to have towards the trauma. Remember what she said when I asked her to come back to the feeling of butterflies and to stay with it. The revelation for her was not so much that the feeling eased when she did, but that she was *able* to stay with the feeling in the first place, even though she didn't want to. As she responded to the Clean questions, feeling the anxiety move deeper down from one energy centre to the next, and noticing the thoughts that came with it, she was making exactly those kinds of mind/body connections that help to release trauma in a way that feels safe. Clean Language was originally developed to work with trauma, but it still needs careful calibration to the client's actual bodymind responses, as well as to your own, to avoid that danger of amplifying the symptoms and the client's understandable anxiety about them.

3.3 WORKING WITH
EMBODIED DOUBLE BINDS

We have all had clients whose problems just won't go away, who are so stuck that some unwanted symptom appears to have become a part of their sense of who they are. We have all been through times like that ourselves. Life repeatedly brings us to these points where we have tried everything to solve some problem and nothing has worked. Maybe we even try accepting that there's nothing we can do about it, hoping that that will make a difference, but it doesn't. The problem is still there, and we usually have a metaphor to describe it: it's like hitting a brick wall, or running round in circles, or a black hole from which no escape is possible. Irony and cynicism become natural companions when we think about such problems, or perhaps we give up thinking about them altogether, seeking out chemical comforts, the reassurance of a doctor's diagnosis, the vicarious reality of virtual worlds or, my own default pattern, attempting to heal or control other people in whom I think I spot the same kind of pattern.

Problems that persist like this are almost always the result of double binds. People usually think a double bind is a situation where you're damned if you do and damned if you don't, but actually that's just a bind, a simple dilemma. For example, say the hero of a movie is clinging to a ledge by her fingertips. If she lets go she will drop into the boiling river of lava below, but if she holds on, her arch-enemy will chop her fingers off one by one. This is a bind, a pretty bad one in fact, but it's still not a double bind. The 'double' refers not just to the 'damned if you do and damned if you don't', but to a second level of the bind that makes it, by definition, impossible to escape, so long as you stay within the logic that the double bind creates.

In movies, characters escape from single binds all the time. Our hero might spot some rocks that she can use as stepping-stones across the lava, let go of the ledge and save her fingers. But say, for example, an evil sorcerer has put a curse on her, so that whenever she finds herself in a bind, she hears a voice in her head telling her that she was never any good at being a hero, and she might as well give up now and join forces with her arch-enemy, who at least seems to believe in what he's doing. Double binds perpetuate themselves so effectively because instead of introducing a new possibility, they do the opposite; they hold their victim in a default pattern of negative self-belief.

One chilling example of this was given by Gregory Bateson, the man who invented the term 'double bind', a brilliant thinker across many disciplines, whose work was a major influence on the development of systems theory and cybernetics. In *Steps to an Ecology of Mind* (1972) Bateson quotes from a chapter in the children's book *Mary Poppins* (Travers 1934/1998), in which she takes her charges to an old sweet shop they have never noticed before. Inside, two sisters, both very miserable young women, are about to serve them when they're interrupted by the brittle, cackling voice of their mother, the sweet shop owner. As soon as she appears, the sisters begin to look nervous and ill at ease. When their mother asks if they've served the children yet, one sister whispers fearfully that they were just about to. At that, their mother flies into a fury and asks who gave them permission to give away her sweets. A tear rolls down the tongue-tied daughter's cheek, at which her mother, shrieking with derision, calls her a coward and a cry-baby.

What makes this a double bind? Their mother is using a classic bully's tactic, keeping her daughters in constant fear that they will be damned if they do and damned if they don't. So far, just a single bind, but a very painful one. On top of that, she has instilled in them the belief that it is all their own fault, that they are cowards and cry-babies with no will of their own. They are disempowered and depressed and can see no escape from their mother's cruelty. If they came to see you for some professional help and you asked them, '**What would you like to have happen?**' they would probably be so caught up in the double bind that you would have to ask them several times in several different ways before they could get any real sense of what a positive outcome would be like, or how to express that in words. So how can we work successfully with double binds?

～ 27 ～

THE PANTHER IN THE CAGE

In this first case study about how to work with double binds, the impossibility of making a choice seems to have become part of the client's way of being in her own body. The first part of the session is a patient but at times frustrating negotiation between the two sides of her body, which seems to be happening entirely at the somatic level. Eventually these two sides of her acquire voices, and the work moves to a more metaphorical level. Only when she finds the key metaphor, the one that seems to emphasise the absolute impossibility of any escape from the manipulative power of the double bind, does something begin to shift for her. As you read it, you will probably find it hard to stay with the many twists and turns of the first part of the session (I have edited that part to about half its real length), but if you do, you'll notice how often apparently meaningless signals from the body do in the end make sense, and how much somatic groundwork you sometimes have to do before any real shift can happen.

A university teacher in her early 30s comes with back pain. She has scoliosis and says that from the age of 10 until 16 her parents insisted that she wear a corset even at night to prevent the scoliosis from getting worse. She was only allowed to take it off for a few hours on hot summer days, and she vividly remembers being able to touch her own skin again on those days. Her hand re-enacts this as she tells me, her fingers lightly touching her upper chest.

Thanks to the scoliosis, she says, the left side of her lower back is 'like stone', and lately she's also had some pain in her sacrum, so I ask:

And which of those are you drawn to most?
- My lower back. Whenever I have trouble with my mother it gets worse. Around my diaphragm, my breath doesn't feel free.

The reference to her mother is tempting, but I don't want to play the amateur psychotherapist, so I keep my next question as open as possible, to see whether it takes us into the relationship or back to the physical sensations:

And is there anything else about all that?
- The left side of my body feels like it has to bear all the weight. The right side feels too weak.

And is there anything else about bear all the weight?
- A friend told me my mother had a narcissistic personality and when I looked it up I found an exact description of the ways she behaves. She is the kind of person who never admits that she has done anything wrong and who makes you feel guilty. When I try to have a rational argument with her, she changes the topic, distorts my own words or just says, 'I can't talk to you; you are unable to understand.' As a child I felt my parents didn't take me seriously. They would laugh at me when I cried, and they never seemed concerned about my feelings. The worst thing was, they would always stick together in opposing their

view of reality to mine, presenting it as the only rational and true one possible, and letting me feel totally wrong and crazy.

And what was that like, to feel totally wrong and crazy?
- My feet don't feel steady on the ground.

After all that narrative, we suddenly come back to a bodily sensation, as if her bodymind wants to get back into the conversation. I suggest that since she is very aware of this imbalance between her left and right sides, we explore first how the two sides of her body feel. She agrees.

And which side are you drawn to most?

She stands up and says the right side feels like it wants more weight. But when I ask if she can gently bring more weight into her right foot, she feels the foot can't take it. I ask her if it would be okay just to stay with that sense that her foot can't take the weight, and she does, shifting her weight slightly more to the right, and what she says next is interesting.

- I'm noticing that the will of my right side to have more weight is stronger than my right foot's sense that it can't take that weight.

She stays with the feeling that the right side wants more weight and after a while finds that the right foot is okay with that. As she shifts more weight into her right foot, she suddenly becomes aware that there is not enough weight in her left shoulder.

What would this left shoulder like to have happen?

She says she doesn't know, so I ask what it's like in her opposite shoulder.

- It's too heavy. It's annoying.

And is there anything else about annoying?
- Like it's trapped in itself. It should open but something is holding it closed.

And where is that holding coming from?

Now she is aware of a knot mid-spine and as she pays attention to it, she says her head starts to feel so heavy that her shoulders feel they need to hold it up.

And then what happens?

Slowly, she lets her head hang down to the front, and gradually feels her right shoulder becoming less heavy and the 'closed' feeling opening up. Then she starts to feel that it's her left shoulder that has 'Too much weight, too much mass,' and at the same time, other parts of her left side are saying, 'We are also too full,' and there's a pain in her lower left side. When she stays with it, it seems to be saying, 'Just relax; I am so tired.'

As the facilitator of this process, at a practical level I'm finding it hard to remember all these different parts of her and their individual needs. At the same time, at the emotional level I'm suspecting that something very important is going on for her in simply allowing all these different parts of herself to be felt. No wonder she's feeling the need to relax.

And can you relax?

She nods. After a while, she says the feeling she started with of the left side having to take all the weight has reversed.

- It's a very strange feeling, as if I could lose my balance and fall to the right. And the right side is afraid it will have to take too much weight, as if it is saying, 'Please do something for me too, not just for the left side.'

Her bodymind seems to be making it very clear that there is some kind of bind at work. As soon as one side gets what it wants, the other side starts to make itself felt. And now she becomes aware again of the old familiar pain in the left side of her back.

- It's been feeling tired and tight for so long, as if it's consumed.

And is there anything else about consumed?
- It's as if it's been resisting for a very long time.

And when it's as if it's been resisting for a very long time, **then what happens?**
- There is sadness. And a narrowness in my breathing.

We have shifted to the emotional level, and maybe a somatic expression of that in this 'narrowness' in her breathing.

And is there anything else about that sadness and narrowness in your breathing?
- My ribs feel like a cage.

And what would your ribs **like to have happen?**
- They want to open.

And can they open?
- It's so entangled inside, it doesn't know how to open.

And what needs to happen when it's so entangled?
- Movement.

But she stays quite still, eyes closed. She seems very internally focused. After a pause, she says:

- It's not an impulse to move physically, it's an image of a lot of cables very tangled up and as if some movement could begin to untangle them.

Then she does have a sense of physical movement: she starts stretching up on one side and down on the other, and then swinging gently round from one side to the other – movements which open the two sides of the body and encourage communication between them.

She has a sense of nausea as she does this, but carries on. As she stretches over to her right side, she feels something stuck in her left side at the waist. In yoga, she says, she usually pushes on through this feeling, putting more effort into the stretch to get through the stuck point.

I suggest she stretches gently up to the stuck point and no further, and just listens to it.

– It feels like it has to hold on, like it's saying, 'I'm doing my duty.'

I ask if she can ease off and then come gently back down into the stretch. She is surprised that she can go much further into it now, and the stuck point feels like it has moved further down her left side. As she stays there and listens to it she says:

– It's quiet there now.

She stretches to the right again, and now says:

– My whole left side is crying out, saying it's very tired.

And when it's very tired, **what needs to happen?**
– It needs to relax and recover.

And can it relax and recover?
– No.

What needs to happen *for it to be able to relax and recover?*
– I need to lie down on my right side.

She does, but after a while, she feels the right side too is saying, 'I'm longing for relaxation but it's not possible.'

And what has to happen *for it to be possible?*
– To have better grounding, and more support from the lower back.

And how would that be?
– A feeling of security; it can let go.

And can it let go?
– It doesn't believe at all that it can have that support.

Now there is a response in the left side. She says the muscle is tightening, and this tightening also has a voice: 'You know you'll never change. Every time you try to change, you fail and just go back to the way you were before.'

Again, I'm tempted to jump in and make a direct connection to what she was saying about her parents earlier, but aware of that, I keep the next question open:

And what kind of voice is that voice?
- It's the voice of despair, and it's consuming me.

There's that 'consuming' again, and coming from the same place – her left side.

Is it a familiar voice?
- Yes, very familiar.

And is there anything else about despair?
- There's a general feeling of being small and defeated and weak.

She collapses her shoulders inwards towards her chest.

And is there anything else about that?
- You burn all the fuel and there is nothing left.

And when all of that, what would you like to have happen?
- Part of me is very pessimistic – you always try to change but it's no good.

And when you always try to change but it's no good, *that's like what?*
- Weakness, narrowness, like an animal in a cage. It wants to get out but the bars are made of iron. It puts all its effort into trying to bite through them but it only harms itself more and more – there is actually no possibility of escaping.

The bleakness of her metaphor makes me pause for a moment, not in doubt but in hope. Perhaps it's pure coincidence, but her image reminds me of Rilke's famous poem 'The Panther', an intense depiction of utter hopelessness (see page 254). Writing it was a huge creative breakthrough for him, and helped him escape the double binds of his own childhood. It's as if by reaching for this metaphor my client is unconsciously communicating that somewhere inside she really does know where this session is going.

I resist the temptation to mention the poem, and instead, I decide to slip out of Clean mode and offer a gentle challenge to that bleak image, by asking if this pessimistic part of her has noticed that she has already made changes successfully in this session. But the pessimistic part isn't interested. After a pause, she says:

- It's like it's in its own reality. I want to ask it, 'Why are you there?'

She gets two answers. One seems to come from her body and says, 'It's for your own good, to protect you. I have to remind you of how the world really is.' The other answer, she says, is 'Like hearing my father talking about "The absolute need of being a realist". It's like I'm hearing his voice and seeing the expression on his face.'

When she says this she feels some movement in her back on the left side, the place where this whole session began.

*And when there's movement there, **what happens?***
- It's like that pessimistic part is saying it needs to be convinced. It needs proof that this reality of my parents is not true.

*And **how** could it be convinced?*
- It says, 'If you never fail in anything, then I will be convinced.'

She says to it that it's not so bad to make mistakes, and actually, it's just not possible to live a life without any failures ever. Then, she says, it goes into a sulk and says, 'I won't talk to you any more, you are crazy.'

Although she has already mentioned her father's voice, she doesn't explicitly identify this new sulky voice as her mother's, even though it sounds exactly like that maternal voice she was talking about at the start of the session. But the connection seems so obvious, I don't feel the need to ask her about it. What's most obvious right now is that we seem to have come full circle, and straight into a wall of uncompromising resistance from these internalised parental voices. But at the same time, this painstaking somatic search for balance between her left and right sides may possibly have laid the foundations for something to shift in her relationship with the voices, which have been so dominant up to now. Again and again, though very cautiously and slowly, her body has been willing to risk doing something differently. The scoliosis seems almost like a physical metaphor for her efforts as a growing girl to find her own truth while being constantly pulled to one side or the other by her parents' impossible demands.

Sometimes, when an internal voice refuses any mediation, the best thing is to call its bluff. So rather than trying to plead with it, I just say:

And since this part won't talk to you any more, I suggest we work directly with the body now, since that is where the change has been happening. Would this be a good point for you to lie down?

She agrees, and as she gets herself comfortable, I say a few words to help us set our intention for the bodywork, talking not just to my client's conscious mind, but also to that part of her that seems to have absorbed her parents' beliefs and behaviour. I explain that no one seems to be happy with this situation, but sometimes things can go on being stuck for a very long time, not because no one wants to change, but simply because no one knows how to change. The aim of using some bodywork is to listen to both sides and to see if there might be something somewhere that's ready to change, since a change anywhere in a system can help every other part of that system.

I sit for a while beside her, and after grounding myself again, I ask her where she would like some touch, using the Clean Touch approach described in Chapter 31.

- My belly.

And what kind of touch would that be?
- A warm, nourishing, physical touch.

I put my hand very gently on her abdomen. It stays there for a long time. Eventually I ask what it's like there now.

- Very relaxing.

I keep asking her for instructions to make sure that the bodywork I'm doing stays as 'Clean' as possible. When there is conflict going on in a system, it's easy to appear to be taking sides, whether you're working with words or with touch. This way at least I know what I'm doing is coming from her own sense of what her body wants. As the treatment progresses, the sense of trust at the somatic level deepens, and I stop asking her for direction and begin to follow where my hands want to go, checking occasionally that that's okay with her.

Two main themes emerge: First is a habitual overactive sympathetic nervous system, with corresponding muscle tension in the back of the neck, the sides of the spine and the back of the legs. The second obvious thing is a real need for grounding, for making a solid contact with the earth. The image comes into my mind's eye of a tree that has grown up on very rocky ground, trying to root itself by twisting and turning from side to side, looking for stability.

I begin to work with the area she said was 'like stone' in her lower back. Gradually there is a response; not exactly a softening, but a willingness to listen. When I ask her what it's like there, she says that the parent part seems very connected with this place in her back. So I ask:

And is there anything else about that parent part?
- It's saying is that under the hardness there is suffering.

And is there anything else about that suffering?
- A crying for love.

And where could *that love* **come from?**
- (She is quiet for a moment) From me.

And can it *come from you?*
- No.

Hearing that 'No', the first thought that flashes through my mind is that maybe she's right: maybe this really isn't going to change, maybe she really is stuck and this whole session has been a waste of time. Then I let the thought go and allow the 'No' to be heard, accepting that there is real truth in it. After all, it's not my response that matters; it's what happens for her when she hears herself say it. And now my hands are feeling a response in her lower back – for the first time in the session, there's a deep sense of relaxation, as if the sympathetic nervous system has finally realised that it doesn't have to be on alert all the time.

I work her left leg and left knee, which hurts at the back. Then the left foot, which needs a warm, confirming touch. Then her right knee, which also feels like it needs a lot of support. These are all ways to encourage the grounding and the sense of solid support that she seems to need so much.

We finish, and I ask her how she is. She says she feels much more centred, and that she really does feel very connected to the earth underneath her. I ask if there's anything else that she experienced during the treatment and she says that at a certain point she asked again that parent part what it wanted and the reply came, 'If you don't need me any more, I'd be glad to go.'

She says this in a very matter-of-fact way, perhaps needing some evidence before she feels safe to trust it. I don't know. But it seems like a very good place to have got to after all that careful work. I'm tempted to ask some more Clean questions about that, but this has already been a very long session so I ask if it's okay to finish there for now, and she agrees.

A couple of months later, she comes for another session and I ask how her lower back is now.

I don't feel it much now. Sometimes the spot is just a little tickly, then the sensation disappears.

*And when the sensation disappears, **what's that like?***
- Freedom. I am free now. I always was free, but didn't know it.

*And when you're free, **then what happens?***
- That critical voice goes away, because actually it never liked to be there either; it was just out of a sense of duty that it stayed there. It says, 'My intention never was to torture you; I just did what I thought I *must* do. I didn't enjoy it, and I will leave you alone if you no longer need me.'

And then what happens?
- It no longer has any power; it was just my parent's thought. Rejecting the parent's thought does not mean rejecting the parent. I have no negative feelings towards the parent.

Interesting that she uses the singular 'parent', without saying whether she is talking about her mother or her father. Maybe the 'parent' has become a kind of generic, archetypal figure. At this point, it seems worth using a different kind of Clean question:

And what difference does knowing that make?
- It's possible for things to change!

She smiles, and it is a joy to see that smile. I suddenly remember that throughout that last session her expression had stayed completely neutral, sometimes with a frown of physical or emotional pain, but never at ease. It was as if her face had been expressing the hopeless disbelief in freedom of that animal in the cage.

And when it's possible...?
- Knowing that opens the way to change. I still have some pain, but it's like after a hurricane. The devastation is still there and it hurts. It takes time to rebuild everything, but the conditions for rebuilding are now ready, and I can feel that it is already starting. I feel my belly getting wider and filling up with energy,

and my breath getting deeper and smoother, and the tension in my back is disappearing.

Notice the change in her metaphors. In the first session, she was an animal trapped in a cage and anything she did to escape just made it worse – a classic symptom of a double bind. Her new 'After the hurricane' metaphor acknowledges the damage and the pain, but now includes the possibility of rebuilding, and she feels ready to do that. When a client makes a real somatic change, their metaphors change too, and asking them to notice that change can not only help them to convince themselves of it, it can also help them to anchor the change symbolically so that they can recall it whenever they need to.

And if somatic change can change a metaphor, the opposite is also true. When you help a client to explore their metaphor, the very act of bringing focused attention to whatever emerges will usually begin a process which involves both sides of the brain and, as we saw so insistently here, both sides of the body. When both mind and body are involved, it can make it much easier for clients to move to that next level of awareness where qualities like compassion and detachment can become part of the equation, releasing the lifelong patterns of a double bind.

THE PANTHER

His gaze is so exhausted from the passing of the bars

that nothing can reach him, or his attention hold.

For him there is only bars

bars without number. Behind them, no world.

That lithe imperious progress, pace by pace

in the tightest of circles cramped and crammed,

is like a spun concentration of pure force

in which a great will is suspended, numbed.

Just sometimes, the covers of the eyes

soundlessly slide open. And into his sight

and taut silence of flesh, an image flies,

only to vanish, forever, in his heart.

Rainer Maria Rilke, translated by Rogan Wolf, 2016

∽ 28 ∽

THE MAN WHO
DESERVED TO DIE

Giving seated shiatsu sessions for a charity at a hostel for homeless men, I go up and down the corridor, knocking on doors, putting my head into the cell-like rooms and asking each occupant if he wants to try a half-hour session. Not many do. One man laughs and says he'd have one if it was a lady doing the massage. Most of these men have been alcoholics for years and are getting too old for the hardships of being homeless in London. They are simply glad to have a room of their own, a TV to watch and the company of other men who know this life and make no judgements.

One day I encounter a man I haven't seen before, sitting on his bed holding a can of diet coke and not doing much of anything as far as I can see. He tells me he has chronic back pain and asks if what I do could help. I say it might. He looks interested for a moment and then says he might try it sometime but he has something else to do this morning. I close the door and move on. This happens again a couple of weeks later, only this time he asks if it could help him sleep better. I say it might. Again, he says he has something he has to do, but might try it sometime. Then one day I hear a knock on the door of my treatment room and it's him, washed and brushed and asking if I'm free.

He sits down in the chair I am using for treatments and we talk about his back pain. He says he's had it for years but it got much worse after a fall a few months ago. I ask if he can feel it now. He says he always feels it, even if he takes the pain pills that the doctor gives him, which he doesn't like to do. I ask if he takes any other medication and he says no. He used to drink but doesn't anymore. He shows me exactly where the back pain is, a little to the left of his lower lumbar vertebrae, and on a scale of one to ten he rates it right now at about five.

I ask if there's anything else. He gives me a quick look, then decides to tell his story. Years ago after a night of hard drinking he got into a fight; the other man fell, hit his head hard on the pavement and died later in hospital. My client says he did his time in prison for this, but still feels terrible guilt for the other man's death, and for the devastation it caused to the man's family and to his own. His wife left him while he was in prison and he hasn't seen his two teenage daughters for some years.

He has one friend who tells him that he's done his time and should be able to put it behind him. 'But everyone else,' he says, 'thinks I should be punished more.' He gestures over to his left when referring to 'everyone else', so I look in that direction and ask:

How do you mean, *everyone else thinks you should be punished more?*
− Like in America – if you kill a man, you have to pay the price.

I ask him how strong his sense is that everyone else thinks he should pay the price. As he thinks about it, he starts swaying very slightly from left to right but doesn't say anything, so I ask:

On a scale of one to ten, if ten is strongest, how strongly do you think that?
− Ten.

And is there anything else about everyone else thinking you have to pay the price?
- I think it's true. It's like karma. Even though I've done a long time inside, I don't think I've been punished enough.

Part of me is wondering if there's anything I can do with Clean Language that could possibly help. Perhaps we should just do some bodywork to help his back. After all, if his belief in his own guilt is that strong, then maybe bodywork and not questions might be the best way to help him feel more at ease with himself. But his bodymind has already given me a clear signal that it knows something about this guilt, and I wouldn't feel comfortable ignoring it, so I ask if he noticed what he was doing when he talked about what everyone else thinks. He didn't, so I imitate the very slight side-to-side swaying motion he'd been making and ask him to do it again. As he does, I point to his left, where he said 'everyone else' was, and ask what it's like there.

He looks a little surprised at first, and then says:

- That's where everybody is who thinks I deserve to die.

This discovery that 'everybody' has such a specific location in his personal space makes him sit up straighter in his chair. Even though he gestured there earlier, the gesture was obviously unconscious, as those gestures usually are. I could ask him more about that left side, but it seems to have such a negative charge to it, as if it is the anchor for his terrible sense of guilt, that I want to find somewhere more positive first. Should I ask him the Outcome question, as a kind of antidote for that negativity, or would that be too much of a challenge too soon? I decide to follow the side-to-side clue his body has already given me. Even though he hasn't mentioned anything about his right side yet, the logic of his movement means there must be something there.

And what happens over there on the right?

- (He tilts his body to the right and thinks for a moment) That's where my friend is, who says I've done more than enough time in prison.

And is there anything else about that?

- He says I should stop blaming myself for it because I never meant to kill him; it was just a fight and I was stronger than the other man.

*And when he says you should stop blaming yourself for it, **what happens** over there on your left where everyone else is?*

- (He leans slightly to his left again, thinking) It's like some of the people over there move around to here…

He holds his hands out in front of him, palm to palm and about a foot apart. Again, he's looking surprised at the way his gestures seem to have a mind of their own.

And is there anything else about the people there in front of you?

- They're kind of neutral about it. They might be people who've had something like that happen to them, so they're more forgiving.

As he says this, his right hand touches the midline of his chest at the base of his sternum and he lets out a little sigh. I nod in acknowledgement of it, but decide to carry on with the investigation of the left and right dynamic rather than bringing his attention to this new gesture yet.

*And when the people there have had something like that happen to them, and they're more forgiving, **what happens** to the people on the left?*

- (He turns to his left again, head down, eyes half-closed, really concentrating now) They start moving a bit more; they're not in such a solid lump; they're moving so there's more space between them.

And when there's more space between them, **then what happens?**
- (He brings his hand back to the spot on his sternum, holding it there this time and letting out another little sigh) They can see my back is killing me, and that I don't drink any more.

And is there anything else about the people over there?
- They know I'm never going to do that again.

And when they know that, **what happens** to the belief that you should be punished more, that you should pay the price?
- It's not the same.

How would you rate it now, when your friend on the right thinks you did more than enough time in prison, and the people there in front are more forgiving, and the people over on your left know that you're never going to be able to do that again?

Here I'm deliberately summarising in a way that stacks all the positive factors on top of each other, hoping that when he hears them all together it will create enough of a charge to shift that old belief that he deserves to die.

- It's sort of going up and down; sometimes it's ten, and then it goes down.

Where does it go down to?
- About seven or eight.

And what's that like when it's seven or eight?

Another sigh, deeper this time, and then silence. He leans forward and looks down, nodding slowly to himself, taking time to process all this. I ask if that would be a good place for me to start working on his back and he says, 'Okay'.

I work gently down his back, exploring the landscape of his whole spine. The muscles where he says the pain is feel tired and empty, but what draws me most is not the lower back but a clenched lump of muscle to the right of his spine higher up, directly opposite the spot on his chest that he had touched before. It's very tight, almost impregnable. Instead of trying to work directly on it, my fingers begin to feel for the weaker spots around it, looking for a way in. At the same time, I use one hand to support his lower back, where the pain is.

After about ten minutes of this, he takes a very deep breath and straightens up. I ask:

What just happened?
- There's something here (he touches the bottom of his sternum again).

What kind of something? **What's it like** there?
- Like I want to breathe in deeper but I can't.

And is there anything else about that?
- Like something's rusted in that won't come out.

And when something's rusted in that won't come out, **what would you like to have happen?**
- I don't know.

As he says this, my fingers on his mid-back feel a tiny spasm in that lump of muscle, and he suddenly lets out a very forceful breath, then breathes in much more deeply than before. The next outbreath is like a spasm through his whole rib cage, and as it comes out, he winces with pain and his hand shoots to his lower back. I ask him how strong the pain is there and he says, 'Ten'. I ask if he can let his breathing come back to normal, and he does. The back pain begins to ease, and I keep my hand there to listen and support.

Meanwhile, I think about double binds. Here is a man who believes that he deserves to die for what he did, or at least a part of him does, and metaphorically, of course, it's his back that has taken over the job of 'killing' him. The Clean questions have already shown him that it is possible to loosen that belief, and his body seems to be showing us both that the feeling of wanting to breathe more deeply is connected with that, loosening whatever it is that's rusted in and won't come out. But if those powerful spasms and gulps of air are an attempt to release that stuckness, they are also triggering the intense back pain. If I carry on trying to release that mid-thoracic lump of muscle, it will probably bring more spasms of deep breathing, which in turn will probably make the back pain unbearable. This is a bind in a physical form, but probably one that would shift with a few shiatsu treatments. But somewhere deeper inside, I imagine, what has held the bind in place for so long is his belief that there's no escape from it, just as he's decided there's no escape from the guilt.

We are at a delicate point, and I'm feeling stuck, which is exactly what double binds do, not just to the client but to the practitioner too. It takes me a minute to realise this, and another minute before I remember that what you do when you feel stuck is to hand that stuckness back to the client in the form of the Outcome question.

And when *you take these deeper breaths, and then your back hurts more,* *what would you like to have happen?*
- For my back to let me breathe.

As he says this, I feel a tightening in his lower back.

And can *your back let you breathe?*
- No. It hurts too much.

Would it be okay if I work on your lower back to see if it could relax enough for you to be able to breathe?

He agrees to this and I begin to work with various points in his lower back. The pain eases off and I take the risk of coming back to that lump of muscle in his mid-back. It's a little softer now so I hold one hand there and support his lower back with the other and ask him to breathe down into the base of his sternum again, but this time to do it gently, breath by breath, feeling for any warning signals from his lower back.

He can do this. He closes his eyes and just continues to breathe. I bring one hand round to the front at the base of his sternum, and keep the other one supporting his lower back. Gradually, the jarring sense of stuckness seems to shift into something more at ease, more peaceful. His eyes are still closed and the expression on his face is more neutral and relaxed, as if he's found a way to be mindfully present with his breath and his back at the same time. His breath gets deeper and deeper until there's a little spasm on the exhalation, but this time it's okay with his lower back. A few more spasms; still okay. I ask him what's happening now.

- I don't know. I'm sorry.

I am holding my hand over his sternum, wondering what he means. Then there is another spasm in his breath and the 'Sorry' comes out this time much louder, almost a sob. He winces slightly but says the pain is okay.

Is he just embarrassed by these strange involuntary breaths, or is he really saying 'Sorry' not to me but to the man he killed? Would it help if I suggest that? Would it help if he asked to be forgiven? How can I keep it Clean?

And is there anything else about sorry?
- I'm sorry to that poor bastard. Like, 'Sorry, mate, you shouldn't have got in that fight.'

*And when you're sorry to that poor bastard, and he shouldn't have got in that fight, **then what happens?***
- This sounds stupid, but it's like he's saying, 'It's alright, I'm okay.' Like he's saying that to me, 'Just fuck off, mate. Just get on with your life.'

*And when he says that, **then what happens?***

There's a long pause. His breathing steadies. I stop doing any active work and just keep one hand on his lower back. I'm wondering if he is feeling what I'm feeling – a powerful current of compassion suddenly melting the space between us, as if for a moment we are no longer two separate people. Eventually, it subsides.

We have already gone way over time, but I need to ask the three things that I always ask at the end of the session. The first one is, 'And how are you now?' He says he's okay. The second one is, 'And was there anything else you noticed during the treatment?' He says the pain in his back was agony, but the feeling of wanting to breathe deeper was even stronger than the pain, so he did. My third question is, 'And with all of that, what happens now when you come back to that place on your left where the people who thought you should be punished more were before?'

He looks to his left and pauses, then says that they're still there, but it's different now.

What kind of different?
-   They're just getting on with their own lives now; they're not so bothered about me.

*And when they're getting on with their own lives now, **then what happens?***
-   Then I get on with mine.

We finish there and I suggest that he have some treatments from an acupuncturist colleague who also visits the hostel; because of other commitments it will be a month before I can come back.

The next time I knock on his door, I find that someone else has taken his room. The supervisor on duty tells me that he has moved out to a room of his own in a house owned by the charity. Apparently this is a kind of upgrade available to hostel residents who are ready to take the next step towards leading an independent life. When I check with the acupuncturist, she says she gave him two treatments and that his back pain has become manageable enough for him to start training for an IT job as part of a re-employment programme run by the charity.

I never saw him again, so I don't know how he rated our session or what he thought it did for him. And I can't say how exactly his back pain was historically related to his need to breathe deeper, or how either of them was related to his belief that 'everyone else' thought he should be punished more. That kind of diagnosis isn't the aim in Clean Language. But I learned a lot about how, if we ask the right questions, we can explore the connections between self-limiting patterns in the body and the beliefs that may be causing them.

Beyond that, all we need to do with Clean questions is to hold the space so that our clients can explore the dynamics of those relationships in the moment. The rest is up to them…and whatever kind of bodywork we have to offer.

~ 29 ~

THE ROOT OF THE PROBLEM
THAT CAUSES THE PAIN

What helped me most in learning to work with trauma and with double binds was realising that both are very natural parts of human experience – no life is lived without them – and that any sense of frustration or hopelessness that arises for the client in confronting them will naturally influence me too. It is easy to feel lost or helpless if I'm trying to guide the client to some hoped-for resolution when they are trapped in a logical framework which offers none. So I am more relaxed about this than I used to be. When I notice myself, as the practitioner, beginning to feel lost or helpless, that is usually enough in itself to allow some new kind of resource into the field between us; and what tells me that a new resource has arrived is that, eventually, I get my sense of humour back. In the following case, while teaching a workshop where I think I am just supposed to be demonstrating how to ask the Outcome question, I find myself working with both a trauma and a double bind. As we've already seen, one of the best antidotes to that potentially toxic combination is the Outcome question itself.

Teaching in Athens, where you could say the word 'metaphor' comes from, I am with Vera, who has agreed to be the subject of a demonstration of how to use the Outcome question. We are standing in front of a group of about 30 shiatsu therapists who are chanting and swaying along to the rhythm of the nine words Vera has just uttered. As we get into the swing of it, I'm realising that the 'carrying across' that metaphors do is not always just verbal or symbolic; here the rhythm itself is the metaphor, carrying across subtle somatic information from the bodymind to the thinking brain.

Vera has offered to be the subject of this demonstration for three reasons. First, she has been suffering from a strange pain in her right shoulder which started four days before the workshop began. Second, she is pretty sure that this pain is caused by the stress of something going on in her life at the moment, and she wants to know – since she knows what the problem is and is doing her best to resolve it – why the pain has not gone away. Third, something very interesting happened yesterday on the first morning of the workshop when I asked everyone to stand up and imagine – just to *imagine* – raising their arms, without making any actual movement. The point of this exercise is to show just how much neurological activity is triggered by thought alone; if you try it yourself you might find sensations of lightness or tingling or simply a heightened awareness of the muscles involved in the movement you're thinking about making.

What Vera noticed was that the level of pain in her shoulder, which since the evening before had been as bad as it could be – a 'ten out of ten' on her own subjective pain scale – had eased off after the imagined movement to something much more bearable, something more like six out of ten. But what happened next was even more interesting. During the break, a technician trying to set up a microphone for us accidentally put a lead into the wrong socket and the whole room burst into a full-powered explosion of white noise, every speaker in this well-equipped studio blasting static into our ears. It was only for an instant, and soon we were laughing it off, but for Vera the shock to her eardrums had brought the pain in her shoulder back to the ten-out-of-ten level it had been before.

Smiling a little nervously, Vera comes up to join me in front of the group. I ask where she would like to sit, where she would like me to sit and where she would like Despina, the translator, to sit. (Vera is happy to speak in English, so the translation is for the rest of the group.) Vera positions us quite carefully; me to her left and Despina slightly behind us; then we begin.

In the edited account that follows, everything I say to Vera and the group is in italic type, and there is also some added commentary for you, the reader, in plain type. Not all my questions to Vera are Clean questions, but when they are, you will see the core parts of each question in bold type as usual.

*Vera, yesterday you had that incident with the microphone – a very sudden, very loud noise. **And then what happened?***
 – I was very scared by it, and the pain came back more strong and I couldn't get back that feeling of less pain I had at the beginning. And then when I got home, I didn't want to have the same night without sleep, so I took some painkillers.

And if we had a scale of one to ten, where ten is the worst possible pain, what was it for you yesterday?
 – Ten – that's the way I felt it.

I repeat Vera's words, 'That's the way I felt it,' and mirror the movement that came just before the words, contracting her right shoulder, tilting her head to the right and tightening her chest. This emphasises that I am listening to Vera's body as much as I am listening to her words, and though both seem to be in agreement at the moment, we will probably get to a point quite soon when they aren't. When that point comes, I want all the non-verbal parts of Vera to know that I'm listening to them just as much as I am to what she's saying.

Your body just gave us an important piece of information. Did you notice the movement you made when you said, 'That's the way I felt it'? On that same scale of one to ten, what's the normal level of pain there in your right shoulder?
-   I think...uh, I don't know why...it comes, 'Three'.

Thank you; it's so important, just to notice that 'I don't know why'. When you ask Clean questions, that's often how the answers come, with this sense of 'I don't know why...but it comes.'

So three is the normal level. **And was there anything else about** *it being at ten yesterday morning?*
-   Yes, it was not only the pain, it was a fear that I can't move and that I can't help myself.

Very understandably, when something is wrong physically, the mind often starts to worry about what the symptom might mean, how bad it might get and so on, and that worry can create its own negative body chemistry and muscle tension, leading to a spiral of anxiety and pain. One way to put the brakes on this pattern is to come gently but firmly back to the '**Where...?**' question, giving anxious thoughts a location which can then make them easier to work with.

And when *there's fear that you can't help yourself,* **where is** *that fear?*
-   Here (Vera points to her chest).

And what's it like there?
-   It's like something suffocating. Not literally, but emotionally. A burden.

Vera has offered us a metaphor; or maybe two – a 'burden' and 'suffocating', and these both seem to relate to her fear that she can't move her arm and that she can't help herself. As I start getting curious about these metaphors, I can also see that Vera is looking quite uncomfortable as she connects with these strong negative sensations in her chest and the metaphors that come with them. Part of me wonders if it would be better to take the pressure off and ask if she'd prefer to carry on our investigation through bodywork, perhaps asking a few more questions as we go. But then I remember that the aim of this demonstration is to show how to use the Outcome question and that we haven't even got to it yet, and suddenly I find myself saying exactly what I need to say to Vera and the group:

Remember the basic principle of Clean Language: it's not that Vera is here for me to fix her; my job is just to help her find whatever she needs to be able to take the next step towards – what?

This may not be the classic form of the Outcome question, but it seems to work because Vera's reply suddenly shifts the session into a different gear.

– Towards the root of the problem that causes the pain.

'The root of the problem that causes the pain,' I repeat, surprised, since her English suddenly sounds fluent: deliberate, decisive and with a rhythm to it that wasn't there in anything she's said so far. As you can see from the next few lines of dialogue, it takes me a little time to grasp the real significance of this.

There's a lovely rhythm to that, as you say it in English. So now we're moving toward the outcome, and Vera's not just saying she wants the pain to go away...
– I want that too! But I know if I do only that, it will come again back.

Yes. So you want to...what was it again?
– To find the root of the problem that causes the pain.

As I repeat Vera's outcome, I find myself tapping out the rhythm, saying it again and again, 'The root of the problem that causes the pain. The root of the problem that causes the pain...'

Vera smiles and the whole group begins to laugh. So do I, but there's a serious point too:

I'm not just joking here. Remember that poetry is one way that language can move from the left brain to the right, and when a client starts to speak with a rhythm, it's just as important a signal as making an unconscious gesture or coming up with an unexpected metaphor. There is a metaphor in this as well – there's a 'root' – and there's a rhythm too: the root of the problem that causes the pain. What is that rhythm like for you? Maybe just stand up and see how your body responds – what starts to happen? Where do you notice it?

Vera stands up and so do I and as she repeats the line she starts to move her hips to the rhythm, shifting her weight from one foot to the other.

– My feet.

And what is it about *your feet?*
– More stable.

And when *your feet are more stable,* **then what happens?**

Vera's movements are already showing us the answer; as she moves her hips and feet to the rhythm of the words, her arms are now swinging freely by her sides, as if the pain is already much less.

– I don't feel so much fear.

And where is *it you don't feel so much fear?*
– I open my chest and my heart.

And what's that like, *when you open your chest and your heart?*
– I feel a little bit better.

And when *you come back to the root of the problem that causes the* *pain,* **what happens when** *you repeat it to yourself as you move?*

Vera repeats it a few times, and starts to laugh.

Workshop demonstrations always have a theatrical element: two people in dialogue, one with a problem, one trying to help; there is the tension of whether or not it will work and the surprise as hidden issues emerge; and above all, there is an audience. All the elements of drama are there, so why not make use of them? After all, we're in Athens, where theatre was once considered to be an essential ingredient in healing the psyche, so when we have a Greek chorus of 30 trained therapists available, why not take advantage? I ask the whole group to stand up and we all start chanting, 'The root of the problem that causes the pain,' clapping and swaying to the rhythm. Led by Vera, we are all laughing now, until she comes back to standing still with her hand on her chest and we all sit down.

And how is it now there in your chest?
– A bit relieved, but I can feel something moving.

And what kind of something moving?
– It's nice but a little – like a tremble...

And is it okay just to stay with it? Just for now, stay with this little tremble?
– It came down.

And what happens next? Take your time, just breathing.

There's a long pause. Vera says nothing but is obviously deeply focused on what's going on inside her. For me it's a welcome opportunity to come back to a sense of simple presence, to let the excitement of the group energy calm down and simply be present with myself and with her.

And what's happening now?
– Now it's calm, and I feel full here (she gestures to her chest), it's okay now.

And how is it when it's okay?
– Peaceful.

And is there anything else about peaceful?
– I'm stable on the ground.

You're stable on the ground. So, all the somatic information at the moment seems to be about a completely different part of the body from your shoulder and arm. It's about your feet and calm and peaceful and stable on the ground.

Is this Vera's bodymind telling us in its own way about the root of the problem that causes the pain? That's just a suggestion from me, so let's go back to asking Clean questions and maybe we'll find out.

And when peaceful, and stable on the ground, where is the root of the problem?
-   It's more here (she indicates her hips and abdomen). But before you asked that, I don't know where it came from, but it came that I can deal with the situation more calmly.

And when it's more there, and you can deal with the situation more calmly, then what happens?
-   I don't know.

Ah – just when I thought we were getting somewhere, we hit a blank. Vera's 'I don't know' sounds to me like it's coming more from her left-hemisphere verbal mind than from that somatic intelligence we've been in dialogue with so far. When this happens it's often a sign that the verbal mind needs time to catch up, or needs proof, or simply needs to be acknowledged.

And what kind of I don't know is that I don't know?

Vera makes a little shrug and says, 'I'll see…' The more light-hearted expression she had just now has disappeared from her face. I think my hunch was right; she needs some proof that whatever we're doing here will be more than just theatre. I slip out of Clean mode to check:

So are we at the point where you feel okay now, but you want to know if it will last, or if something else might happen like that microphone sound yesterday and take it all away again?

Vera nods, wincing slightly as my suggestion brings back the memory of the noise.

Now let's remember that very interesting question Vera was asking yesterday – why do her symptoms persist when she's well aware of the problems in her life that seem to be causing them?
- Yes, why when I know, or I'm almost sure, what the problem is that causes the pain, why is the pain still here? Is it something I haven't seen yet?

*I don't know. But we're making progress. We know more about the root of the problem now. **And when** it's peaceful and you feel more grounded **then you have a sense that...?***
- I can deal with it.

You can deal with it. And here again we can measure; how strong is that sense that you can deal with it?
- And it comes again, three.

*So let's say thank you to wherever three came from, and come back to the Outcome question. **And when** you can deal with it and it's about three, **what would you like to have happen?***
- To get it a bit bigger than three.

***And can** it get bigger than three?*
- Yes.

***And what needs to happen** for it to get bigger than three?*
- (Long pause...) It came: the feet.

***And what is it about** the feet?*
- I feel like I have my feet on the ground and that makes me still all over my body.

Can we do that standing up?

We stand up and Vera does indeed look more stable as she stands there.

And is there anything else about *feet on the ground, stable and I can deal with it?*

As I say this, for the first time in the session I start to feel a real movement of energy coming from Vera – as if her energy field is expanding and giving her more power. But when I mention this to Vera and the group, she immediately notices a negative reaction.

- Now I feel a bit weak…numb in my foot.

Is that a familiar feeling? The numbness in your foot?
- No.

And when you just stay with it, how is that numbness now?
- I feel a bit weaker.

And where is *weaker?*
- Just here (she gestures to her left hip).

So here's an interesting thing. When you're sitting down, the clear message is that your feet need to be on the ground, and as soon as they are, there's numbness and weaker. This can be a frustrating place to get to, so let me just say, Vera, that all we're doing here, carefully and patiently, is getting the structure of this whole pattern, just mapping it out. Not trying to change it, just patiently welcoming whatever comes next and putting to one side the natural professional sense we might have as bodywork therapists of, 'Oh, that's where the pain is so I'll start the treatment.' Sooner or later we'll get to that point.

The purpose of using Clean questions like this is to get to the point where we don't need to ask them any more, where all that's left to work with is the body itself, where the client has done all they need to do consciously, and they can lie down and spend some time in a different state – call it rest or trance or alpha waves or what you like – it's the place where deeper work is being done, work that the left brain may not have language for, and work that as a therapist your hands may know more about than your head. But while we're still working with words, Vera is allowing the hidden pieces of her inner landscape to emerge, and there's still so much happening for her, it would seem wrong to interrupt. When we get to a difficult part of the landscape, the thing to do is to remember what came before, and go back to parts that we've already found have resources to offer. For example:

Is there anything else about the root of the problem?
- Ah! I forgot about that already!

What happens when you re-introduce that resource? When there's numbness and there's weaker and you bring this rhythmical movement to it. The root of the problem...

Vera repeats it to herself, this time more slowly but with the same swaying rhythm in her body.

And what happens when you have that rhythm?
- I smile, first of all...when I listen to it, and the numbness is going away from the right foot and it comes to the left foot!

She laughs loudly as if that is some kind of joke.

And when the numbness moves to the left foot, what happens next?
- It's almost gone.

And when it's almost gone, and the root of the problem that causes the pain, then what happens? What's happening there now? (I point to her chest area.)
- It opens, but I still feel a bit of a burden.

And then what happens?
- It gets stronger.

And now let's bring in another resource – the one that made the difference in the first place. If it's okay, just closing your eyes, coming back to the breath and just imagining the rhythm without actually moving the body...

Here I'm asking Vera to go back to that exercise from yesterday which worked for her so well, just imagining the movement without actually making it. There's another long pause…

How is it down there **now?**
- More familiar.

And what's it like when it's more familiar?
- There's a word but I can't remember it, it doesn't come.

And when it's familiar, and there's a word that doesn't come, **is there anything else about** a word that doesn't come?
- It's like something that can come to give me strength, but it's like I don't want it to come and give me strength.

Now we really are getting to the root of the problem. The resource she needs is there but some part of her doesn't want it. When things get complicated like this it's useful to remember how simple Clean questions really are.

And where is the 'I' that doesn't want it to come and give you strength?
- This part here. Vera points to her chest and sighs.

And now, for the first time in this whole process, I get the sense that Vera's bodymind is communicating directly with me, saying 'Come here, come here,' and drawing my attention urgently to her lower back. For me, this is how the bodywork part of a session begins – when the client's qi invites me in, and not before. But when it does, I need to explain that to the client's conscious mind and make sure that it's okay with them. Holding my hand with my palm towards her, I explain what's happening and ask Vera if it would be alright to put my hand there, since that's what her energy seems to be asking me to do.

- Yes.

So I'm just acknowledging, following with my hand, not trying to do anything, just the sense that there needs to be support there. And

Vera, do you know the basic qi gong standing position, bending the knees slightly so that the curve of the lower back straightens out?

For me this posture does for the body what Clean Language does for words. When you put yourself in this position, you remove many of the body's habitual distortions and make it as easy as possible for the bodymind to listen to itself without any interference. I show Vera what I mean and make sure she can feel her lumbar curve gently straighten and relax.

–   That's weird. Before I did that, the numbness was here again, and when I did that it was gone.

And coming back to your chest, **how is it now?**
–   Lighter.

And when it's lighter, **what happens to** *the something that can come and give you strength, and to your sense that you don't want it to?*

This is a pivotal question, since I've done my best to respond to exactly what I felt Vera's energy was telling me to do, and the signal seemed a very powerful one. If the part in her chest is still not convinced, we may have more work to do, and as far as this demonstration goes, time is running out. There's another long pause and then Vera says:

–   There's no answer.

That's okay – sometimes when there's no answer, something deeper than words is happening.

That wasn't a very Clean thing for me to say, was it? Maybe there is some kind of double bind at work here, and as the practitioner, I am sharing Vera's sense of being trapped by it. When you're a bodyworker in a situation like this, it's worth remembering something Carl Jung is supposed to have said: 'Often the hands will solve a mystery that the intellect has struggled with in vain,' I remind myself to trust my hands. They say that there is indeed something still happening at a deeper energetic level, and that all Vera needs is a little reassurance to stay with it. So I ask her:

Is it okay just to follow your breathing for a minute? Meanwhile my hand is still here connecting with your lower back and I feel something good happening, like the energy is going down. If you want to help that process you could just remember the grounding, and the word that doesn't come...

- Now I feel like I almost don't feel anything, except a little tremble on my knee.

*So let's come back to the Outcome question – **and when** there's a little tremble on your knee, **what would you like to have happen?***

- To be more stable.

And can *you be more stable?*

- Yes.

And what do you need *to be more stable?*

- To breathe deeper.

And what happens *when you breathe deeper?*

As I ask this, I feel a powerful movement of energy in her lower back.

And what just happened?

- Something...

*And here's a new thing...**what kind of something?***

- In my back.

Is it an okay something, or not okay?

- It's okay.

And how is it now?

- It's gone.

There's another long pause as Vera stands, eyes closed, focusing on her breath and on what's going on inside. Meanwhile, I tell the group what's happening for me:

So I'm just testing; can my hand come away from Vera's back yet? It still wants to stay there, but a long way off the body, so my sense of it is that Vera's energy still wants a little help from me but not so much. I feel all my body quite okay...(pause)...except my right calf.

And just come back into your qi gong position, and touch your lower back with your own hand.

There's another pause as she puts her hand on her lower back and stands there a little longer.

***And how is** your calf now?*
 – It's okay.

Notice how painstaking it can be to deal with all the objections that apparently arise when some kind of major shift occurs. First the chest, then the tremble on the knee, then the feeling in the calf. But paying attention to each one in turn helps to ensure that the system will not just snap back into the old pattern that was causing the pain.

*So, Vera, we've got a lot of information now, and **is that an okay place to stop** and sit down?*
 – Yes.

*And let's take a moment to bring this all together for Vera, and for ourselves as practitioners to think about what's happened. The first thing was your outcome; to find the root of the problem that causes the pain. **So how is that now?***
 – I think I am in the beginning. I touch something. And a strange thing – I always need someone to help me, someone stronger. Okay, I am strong, but I need someone to be there for me. But when you asked me to put my own hand there on my lower back it was like I found what gives me that strength.

So no wonder I felt that signal so strongly from your lower back; the strength you were looking for was already there in you.

- I don't know exactly what has happened in this whole process; I just know that whatever came in my mind I said.

It sounds like Vera's cognitive mind is asking to be acknowledged again, which is as it should be, since as soon as the workshop is over it's that cognitive mind which will be in charge again, so I say:

I don't know exactly what's happened either, but there's one more thing we need to do and that's to find out what agreement you can make between your normal everyday cognitive mind and your bodymind about what you want to take away from this; and what you might do differently from now on. What is one thing you'd like to remember from this experience?

- (Smiling) The root of the problem that causes the pain.

And how is the pain now, on that one-to-ten scale?

- Almost one.

And is that a good place to finish this demonstration of how to ask the Outcome question?

- Yes.

Thank you very much, Vera.

Thinking about it afterwards, I realised how many times Vera had, consciously or unconsciously, given us clues that her sympathetic nervous system (her fight/flight response) was deeply involved in all this. Fear was the very first thing she mentioned – 'I was very scared by it, and the pain came back more strong' – and she signalled it again when she talked about her 'Fear that I can't move and that I can't help myself.' The microphone incident was another clue since hearing can become very sensitive in that state of heightened alertness. It's also strongly associated, at least in my own meridian-based approach, with the fight/flight response and with the lower back, the place where Vera finally found the strength she'd been looking for.

Step by step, in response to the Clean questions, Vera's system was showing her how to relax that habitual fight/flight response.

The first step took her down to her feet and the feeling of being more grounded and stable. The second was a sense of opening around her heart. The third was to relax her lower back. With all three of these powerful resources in place, it was much easier for her cognitive mind to challenge that habitual thought she mentioned near the beginning that 'It was not only the pain, it was a fear that I can't move and *that I can't help myself*' [my italics], and to start thinking in new ways. Her old belief – 'I always need someone to help me, someone stronger' – suddenly turned into a new one when she touched her lower back and found that 'the one that gives me the strength', could be herself.

We exchanged a few emails three months later when I sent her the transcript of this session. Her replies reassured me that the movements of energy and the psychological insights she'd experienced weren't just a temporary fix or a theatrical response to the attention of the group. In her first email she said, 'I am very moved right now, because reading our session again, after all this time, it's like something changed inside. Don't ask me what. That, I don't know.' In her second, she said, 'I am much better. My arm is okay with a slight pain now and then. I sing a lot, 'The root of the problem that causes the pain', and I do little steps on supporting myself.'

I asked Vera what had happened with those emotional issues she had mentioned – the ones she thought were causing the pain. She said:

> I don't know exactly what changed with my emotional problems, but I feel the difference in my everyday life. Also I understand now that my emotional problems are a lot more than the ones I thought I had! But it's okay. I ask Clean questions, and I feel that when something changes in my body after a conscious work on it, something changes in my mind, my emotions, my energy and in fields that I am not aware of at the moment. And now and then I feel a pinch of pain. That tells me that I have still things to see. And I am glad that I am able to do that now.

Finally, in answer to a question from me about what it had been like to have the whole group chanting with her, Vera said that at first she felt a bit shy but then, 'I felt energy moving like it was not me, like it was almost freedom.' It is interesting that she hadn't even mentioned that at the time, and interesting too that in writing that sentence in her email she actually made a spelling mistake (the only one she made in all of her four emails to me), and one which seems like a wonderful postscript from that unconscious intelligence that had been guiding the whole process. Writing that she felt a bit shy, Vera had written, 'I felt a *beat* shy' – a perfect way to acknowledge how the *rhythm* of her own words was the invitation to finding the root of the problem that causes the pain.

3.4 HOW CLEAN SHOULD I BE?

However Clean you aim to be with the questions you ask, you are always influencing your client in some way just by being you, by the natural qualities of your voice, your height, your weight, the habitual expressions on your face, the clothes you wear, your cultural background and beliefs, and the intentions you have for yourself and your clients. You cannot *not* influence them, after all, and that obvious truth was brought home to me in a very unexpected way quite early in my shiatsu career on a visit with some colleagues to a complementary health fair.

On one of the stands we noticed something that had the audacity to call itself a 'shiatsu machine' – a white and silver contraption of metal, fabric and plastic, contoured to fit, more or less, any human neck. We were half-amused and half-annoyed by it. The idea that a machine could do something which, as far as we were concerned, was by definition all about human-to-human contact, seemed ridiculous. We had a laugh and soon moved on, but as we wandered among the many stands, I felt a strange curiosity to go and try it out. I found my way back, and once the saleswoman had shown me how to switch it on, I was soon settling into a comfortable chair, feeling the steady mechanical rhythm of the machine's padded rollers on my neck. As I began to relax into it, I noticed a subtle sense of relief – not just physical but something else; what was it?

I could tell that there were a lot of things the machine couldn't do – it felt so impersonal and robotic – but at the same time I realised that the relief I was feeling came from the simple fact that this machine had absolutely no personal issues of its own. For a moment, that sense of not having to connect in any way with another human being was pure bliss. I had never really noticed before, when I had a treatment with a human practitioner, what an enormous amount of energy I unconsciously invested in judging whether I felt safe enough with this person to be able to let go. With the machine, none of that was necessary and it felt so different.

And the real difference was that, alone with myself, in a space uncluttered by any other human presence, there was nothing else to think about but my own sensations. The machine was simply reflecting back to me feelings that were already there inside me, but doing it without any judgemental remarks or diagnostic intentions; like a true master, it had no attachment to what it was doing or how I would respond. This simple sense of freedom from any kind of therapeutic relationship, except the one I had with myself, allowed me to notice one of my most fundamental relational patterns – an over-zealous sympathetic nervous system anxiously patrolling my physical and energetic boundaries. That little machine gave me the space I needed to notice that, a space I remember to this day.

30

CLEAN AND THE THERAPEUTIC RELATIONSHIP

Is that why I was so attracted to Clean Language when I first encountered it? I don't know, but by offering clients a space of their own, it seemed a valuable counterpoint to the closeness of connection that is essential to shiatsu and many other forms of bodywork. Space is by definition closely shared in touch-based forms of bodywork, and the intimacy of touch, so powerful that it is a strict taboo in most forms of psychotherapy, is – in shiatsu, at least – the essential medium of the work.

As Akinobu Kishi and Alice Whieldon explain in *Sei-Ki, Life in Resonance* (2011, p.68), shiatsu's Japanese lineage includes the idea of 'Ai no teate' – a 'therapy of love'. Shizuto Masunaga (Masunaga and Ohashi 1977), whose shiatsu sessions – like love – could sometimes be agonisingly painful, and who pioneered the style of shiatsu which has become most popular in the West, was actually very influenced (to the dismay of his professional peers in Japan at the time) by the American psychologist Carl Rogers and the client-centred approach Rogers developed, fundamental to which is an attitude of 'unconditional positive regard' towards the client.

Clean Language, by contrast, is not client centred. As Philip Harland points out in his book on Clean Language in psychotherapy, *Trust Me, I'm the Patient* (2012, p.128), the primary focus of the Clean approach is not the therapeutic relationship between client and practitioner, but the relationship between the client and their own internal landscape. In technical terms, it's not 'client centred', but 'client information centred', and the practitioner's role is not primarily to help the client understand and come to terms with their past, or even to understand the client at all, but to help them build a rich and dynamic model of that internal landscape, discover its hidden resources and make the connections that create in-the-moment insight and the healing power that brings.

The Clean approach is thus the opposite of the very client-centred focus of most forms of bodywork therapy; in Eastern terminology, the two form a perfect combination of Yin and Yang, in which the well-researched importance of the therapeutic relationship is countered and complemented by an approach in which the therapist turns into a more detached 'facilitator', allowing the client a deeper relationship with their own internal landscape of thought, sensation and feeling, rather than having the therapist interact with and interpret it for them.

What does this mean in practical terms as you explore how to integrate Clean questions into the kind of bodywork you do? Though the questions themselves are simple, learning how to weave them into your work as a practitioner takes a lot of experience – for example, learning how to adjust the style and amount of Clean Language to each particular client, or knowing when to let go of Clean questions completely in the interests of the therapeutic relationship, and how to re-introduce them gently and gracefully into the conversation without manipulating that relationship. For instance, if you treat your client's keywords as something you can improve on or reframe, or if you ask a question which suggests in some way that their view of the world is just plain wrong (both of which could work well as interventions in other kinds of therapy), in Clean Language you're more likely to notice a loss of connection with your client and, even more important, a sense of derailment of their internal process.

In the interview section later in the book, practitioners of various bodywork therapies describe how they manage the delicate business of introducing Clean Language into their work, and the different ways that clients may respond. Going into Clean mode too soon, or failing to get your client's permission, can temporarily rupture the therapeutic relationship and if that should happen it's important not to try to bulldoze through your client's natural resistance by asking more Clean questions (for example, '**And when** you don't understand the question I just asked, **what kind of** don't understand **is that?**'), but to acknowledge the problem and explain how Clean questions can help your client to get more from the bodywork.

CLEAN FOR TEENAGERS

And as well as talking *explicitly* about how Clean Language can help, it's also important to show *implicitly*, in the way you ask Clean questions, that you're flexible and sensitive to how your client responds to them. This is always a step-by-step process of trial, error and negotiation. Here is an extreme example, but one which will be familiar to any parent of a teenager, in which I use a pinch of Clean Language in an attempt to start a conversation with my teenage daughter.

I am concerned because she's looking stressed and rather pale and very preoccupied with whatever is going on in her head. She is working very hard preparing for her exams and has probably been up most of the night. We are in the kitchen, mid-morning, our backs to each other. I am making coffee and she is cutting up a mango for her breakfast. I ask:

What do you have to get done today?
– Stuff (in a mumble, without looking up).

What kind of stuff?
- Stuff.

This time she says it more emphatically, as if it is a genuinely helpful elaboration on her last answer. I decide that any further attempt by me to ask Clean questions will sound to her like Dad is trying his therapist routine and will get us nowhere. So I just give her back what she has given me:

Stuff stuff.

This may sound quite Clean but it's not. In fact, it's my way of saying, 'Do you want to talk to me or not, because I'd like to talk to you?' In response she says:

- Compiling.

Even though what she's offered sounds like a very small nugget of information, to her it may seem like everything I need to know.

Compiling what?
- Art.

Okay, I know it must be art that she's compiling, because art is what she's studying, but she has made a concession and told me something, so now I need to make a concession too. Instead of asking, 'What kind of art?', I need to do a bit more of the work myself. I offer her a choice:

Like what to put in and what to leave out?
- Yeah. It's too many decisions. I think I'm getting ill from the stress.

Suddenly her tone has changed. In my role as 'Dad' this feels like a gratifying shift in our relationship. I want to be a good dad, so I am focusing on the 'therapeutic relationship' aspect of the conversation. To her, the more important shift is probably just noticing how she is actually feeling. The relationship she is focusing on is her relationship with herself.

How do you feel ill?
- I've got a headache, and my head feels slightly warm.

Now we are having a conversation, one in which we can be equal partners and choose what roles to play. I could come back to Clean questions as a way to help her explore her symptoms, or I could ask her about her work, or I could offer some suggestion, or I could just listen and see what else she wants to say.

Whatever kind of response you get when you introduce Clean Language to your clients, you will soon notice certain patterns emerging among them. My simple rule-of-thumb is to think of it like triage: some of your clients will hate Clean Language and would rather go on suffering all their problems than answer a single Clean question; some will take to it immediately and, with very little help from you, will be amazed at the power of the Outcome question and how much their symptoms have to tell them; and most will, like my teenage daughter, need a little coaxing and a lot of flexibility from you before they discover in their own personal way just how useful Clean Language can be.

FACILITATIVE LANGUAGE: QUESTIONS OR SUGGESTION?

Another way to manage this balance between the therapeutic relationship and Clean Language is simply to ask the questions in a different way, or not to ask questions at all. Clean Language exists at one end of the spectrum of facilitative language, the language used by therapists, teachers and coaches to facilitate their clients in any kind of self-exploration process. This language varies from one discipline to another, and from one practitioner to another. One practitioner may sound quite directive, speaking – however gently – in simple commands (for example, when a yoga teacher is telling her students to move into a certain pose), while another may prefer to suggest or invite, switching from the imperative ('And now, do this') into the continuous present ('And now, *doing* this...'). For example, in a mindfulness class, instead of telling the participants, 'Now bring your attention to your breathing,' a teacher would be more likely to say something like, 'Now *perhaps bringing* your attention to your breathing.'

Subtle shifts of language like this can change the whole tone of your communication, implicitly demonstrating to the client that you're flexible enough to move back and forth between the roles of therapist and facilitator, or teacher and coach, depending on what your client seems most comfortable with. If you're interested in exploring the many ways you can use facilitative language, one of the best authorities to consult is the Focusing teacher and innovator Ann Weiser Cornell. A graduate student in linguistics when she met Eugene Gendlin at the University of Chicago in the 1970s, she went on to get her PhD in linguistics while learning and later teaching Focusing. Her books, *The Power of Focusing* (1996), *The Radical Acceptance of Everything* (2005) and *Focusing in Clinical Practice* (2013), have made her a leading figure in the field. In them she brings her linguistic sensibilities to the practical business of sitting with a client and trying to find the right kind of language that will help that unique individual to find their own way into a 'felt sense'. She calls her own facilitative style 'Presence Language', emphasising that the most essential quality you bring to that encounter as the therapist is not the language patterns you use but your ability, in Gendlin's words (1990, p.205), 'to be a human being, with another human being'; she also combines her academic understanding with a personal passion about the role of language in body-oriented therapy. She discusses in depth the benefits of framing your interventions as suggestions or invitations, and lists the many variations you can use to 'cushion' the impact of anything you say, for example using phrases like 'You might...', 'See if it would be okay to...' or 'Take some time to...'

Interestingly for followers of the Clean approach, she strongly questions the value of questions. They are conversationally much more powerful (in the sense of manipulation) than suggestions in both a cognitive and a relational sense, she says. Relationally, they run the risk of bringing the client out of their internal focus and back to an awareness of the interpersonal connection with the therapist. Cognitively, since asking a question presupposes that there must be an answer, when clients are being invited to explore the unfamiliar terrain of the bodymind, direct questions are more likely to get responses like 'I don't know' or 'Nothing', while softer suggestions to simply engage with the process put less pressure on the client to come up with a specific answer.

For example, if your client says they have a pain in their shoulder, and your first attempts to ask Clean questions fail to produce any somatic response, you might switch into a different style of facilitative language:

And where exactly is that pain in your shoulder?
- (The client replies by pointing to the top of their left shoulder blade) That's where I usually feel it.

And can you feel it now?
- No.

And what kind of pain is it when you do feel it?
- I don't really know. I can't feel it right now.

The Clean questions seem to have reached a dead end. There may even be a hint of frustration between you as the client wonders why you're asking these questions. What can you do? One way out that Cornell suggests is to offer the client some choices here, as I did with my teenage daughter; for example:

Is it a sharp pain, or more like an ache?
Is it near the surface or deeper inside?
Does it feel like a muscle or more like it's in the joint itself?

These questions help you to gather more information and they may result in the client becoming more aware of what is actually going on in their shoulder. If they don't, you might ask if they'd like to try a little experiment, and switch from questioning to inviting or suggesting:

*Maybe just **settling down** in your chair for a moment, and **being aware** of the feeling of breathing, and then when you're ready, **bringing your attention to** your shoulder and **noticing what happens**...*

If they still have no in-the-moment sense of something happening in the shoulder, you could simply note that and move on to the Outcome question. Alternatively, you could try one of the most effective body awareness techniques – contrasting the problem area with another part of the body – for example, suggesting to your client that they switch their attention to the other shoulder. So, asking if it would be okay to try another little experiment, you say:

And now letting go of** that left shoulder **and bringing your focus of attention to** the right shoulder, **and just noticing what it's like there.
 - The right one's okay. That's not the problem. It's...actually, it's feeling a bit hot there – that's weird; I never felt that before, hot and kind of twitchy.

At last there's some kind of response from the bodymind, and the process begins...

Personally – having studied both Clean Language and the more invitational language patterns of Mindfulness-Based Cognitive Therapy – I often find myself shifting back and forth between questions and suggestions during any particular session, depending on...well, depending on what? I don't know exactly. Ah, there's that 'I don't know' that she's talking about – I asked myself a direct question and couldn't find an answer. But if I stay with that 'I don't know', then what happens? (Another direct question.) What happens is I start to realise that the shifting back and forth between questions and suggestions that I do with a client seems to be a response to fine-tuned variations in what is going on with my client's face, voice tone, gestures and qi (apologies for importing a technical term from my own field, but I don't know how else to say it) and with my sense of the qi in the field between us.

Of course, you can translate almost any Clean question into a suggestion simply by adding a few words like 'And noticing...' at the beginning:

And noticing what kind of weird that is.
And noticing where exactly that hot and twitchy feeling is.
And just noticing what happens when you ask that shoulder **what would it like to have happen.**

Whether you prefer the directness of Clean questions or the more invitational (and, some might say, even more trance-inducing) language of suggestion, the most important thing is simply to be constantly sensitive to what is working for your client. Clean Language puts you into a space where it is easy to see the immediate effects of any mistakes you make, since there is so little else going on there to distract you. For example, if your client's response to something you say is to turn towards you or make direct eye contact with you, then you have brought them out of their internal focus and back to focusing on you, the practitioner.

In her typically observant and nuanced style, Ann Weiser Cornell mentions an experience she had once as a client in therapy, which is a useful cautionary tale about the problems of over-directive language. In this case, the therapist's question breaks the rules of pure Clean Language twice, first by specifying a particular sense ('feel'), and second, by specifying a particular location ('in your body'). But what Cornell objects to is simply the question itself, which just doesn't work for her until she puts it into her own more invitational language:

> I had a therapist who asked me questions when she intended to facilitate process. Every time she said something like, 'How does that feel now in your body?' I forgave her, translated what she said, and sensed into my body. But there was always a little pang, a little bump. Yes, I could do it myself. But how nice it would have been to just sink deep, undistracted, invited by the words of the guide into gentle and intimate relationship with my own being. (Cornell 2005, p.181)

That last sentence is perhaps one of the best descriptions of the kind of experience that David Grove intended the client to have when he was developing Clean Language. Whether you achieve it by asking questions or by making suggestions, or by a sensitive combination of both, the main point is to do it in that wonderful spirit of detached facilitation that taught me so much when I experienced it from the shiatsu machine at the health fair. In the next chapter, the traditional idea of the therapeutic relationship is challenged even further as we look at 'Clean Touch', a way to use Clean Language in relation to the body that explicitly puts the client in charge of the whole process.

∼ 31 ∼

CLEAN TOUCH

I'm lying on the floor, with a lot of other people similarly supine, in a workshop led by Jackie Calderwood and Jeni Edge, two therapists who met while studying Clean Language. Discovering they shared a background in bodywork, they asked themselves, 'What would it be like to apply Clean principles to the actual process of working with touch?'; not just to ask Clean questions before and after the hands-on work, but to use them throughout the treatment, and not simply as an added ingredient but as the core of the whole process. In other words, instead of assuming you (or your hands) know what the client needs, and using your expertise to provide that for them, you put that expertise aside and agree with your client that they will be the person who guides the treatment, simply by answering your specifically tailored Clean questions.

I'm already familiar with the idea of asking the client to lead the process, since one of my teachers, Bill Palmer, has used it for decades as one of the key ingredients of his experiential bodywork approach known as Movement Shiatsu. It's also used in other forms of bodywork and body-psychotherapy as a way of exploring the relationship between the therapist, the client and the client's bodymind. So what might be different about the Clean version?

Hoping to find out, I am here on the floor with no idea what will happen, especially since the group is fairly evenly divided between professional bodyworkers and people who have little or no experience of working with touch. But after the usual introductions and ground rules, the first exercise is beautifully simple and very reassuring. Making sure we're comfortable and that we've had a chance to tune in to ourselves, Jackie says, 'Ask yourself where would your body like to be touched.' For me, at least, the answer is obvious – only a few weeks before, I broke my wrist and needed an operation to re-set the fracture. As soon as she asks the question, I'm immediately aware (though I hadn't been before) of a kind of dense pulsing ache around the titanium-stapled bone of my right forearm. But the next question is a surprise. 'And what *kind* of touch would this part of you like to receive?' The question makes me realise that I actually have a relationship with this bone of mine. What kind of touch indeed? How would I know? How would it know? My bone, I mean. The answer begins to formulate, less quickly this time, and not in words but as an image in my mind's eye, of a location a few inches above my wrist.

The kind of touch it wants is not physical, not a hand wrapped instinctively round an injured limb, but an 'off-the-body' touch, as if there's something in the energy channels there that, pre-occupied with post-op physio, I haven't got around to noticing. I'm still wondering where this touch is going to come from when Jackie asks, 'And which hand would like to give this touch?' There is a moment of relief as I realise that she's not asking us to work with someone else, that I don't have to surrender this intimate little relationship that's developing between my bone and me to a third party, at least not yet. Also I notice just how much subtle power there is in asking these kinds of questions. Even though logically it would have to be my left hand that would like to give the touch, since it's my right wrist that's injured, the suggestion that there might be a choice seems in itself to spark some intuition inside me. Since my fracture, my left hand has had to work much harder and do many things it's not used to doing. The question slows me down and takes me into a half-dreaming state where I can listen to what my body knows, allowing my awareness to shift back and forth from left to right the way a needle guides the thread that stitches up a wound.

I lift my left hand so that the palm is hovering above and tuning in to the pulsing of my still-swollen right wrist. It feels good to do this. There's no change in my wrist, but I notice a tiny shift inside my chest, as if something can relax there now; as if something there is pleased to be acknowledged. What kind of something? I start to wonder, but Jackie's next suggestion calls me back: 'And explore what happens between your hand and that touch.' I explore. My wrist begins to feel not like a wrist but like an injured animal, as if it's still in shock, confused. Very slowly, my left palm begins to sink down towards it, until I feel the softest hint of contact between left hand and right wrist. This feels good too – acknowledging, reassuring, connecting, listening. The fingers of my right hand start to tingle, as if something is flowing through my wrist, something that was blocked before. 'And is there anything else about that touch...?' asks Jackie.

Of course there is; there's nearly always something else when you're asking Clean questions, as I am about to find out when we start to work with a partner. But let's return to that once you know a bit more about how Clean Touch began and what it's all about. That was the question I put to Jackie and Jeni in an interview after the workshop.

What makes Clean Touch so different from most hands-on therapies?

JE: The way it combines metaphor with touch. One definition we have for what we're doing is: 'Accessing the body's wisdom through metaphor in a shared dialogue of giving and receiving touch'. It's not about me as a therapist getting a client to a particular solution: it's about me facilitating them to have more insight, more understanding, more connection with their own process, so it's a really different way of formulating that relationship with the person you're working with; it's about stepping out of that expert role.

JC: In fact, it's quite useful to ask what Clean Touch is not – it's not a redundancy of expertise, it's a shift in the kind of expertise I might want to develop, perhaps an expertise in what not to be, or how not to be.

JE: Yes, for me there's still a desire to be an expert, but an expert facilitator rather than an expert therapist. I can't imagine now doing a massage session as I used to do them, saying, 'We're going to start off with you lying on the couch, then I'm going to put the oil on,' and so on. In a way that's a lovely thing to do and it has a whole ritual to it, but to me Clean Touch is much more interesting. I find it easier to do, and I actually find it easier on my body too. That's partly from not holding that space of thinking, 'I'm this expert massage practitioner who embodies rhythm and serenity.' Actually, it's about me being me, and knowing when to leave myself out of their process; I'm not trying to solve problems any more, I'm allowing the other person to do that. It's just a completely different way of being and operating.

What gave you the idea for Clean Touch?

JC: It grew out of our wanting to bring what we were discovering from using Clean questions in our massage work into something we could offer in a workshop setting, working through clothing, in a safe environment, with people who might not have a background in bodywork. We're really careful to make the workshop a safe space and to think about possible objections, for example when we have people from both psychotherapy and from bodywork.

JC: And that informs our dialogue when we're working out how to present the material so that people will be comfortable with it and able to learn it easily whatever their background. So it's coming from quite a reflective practice, and a research practice, with an academic rigour and a psychotherapeutic and an ethical rigour too.

The word 'Clean' in Clean Touch doesn't just mean that the client guides the way that touch is used; it's also there as a reminder that when you bring someone's awareness to an embodied issue through questions or touch, the mind often responds in metaphor. But not always. A person may feel comfort, vulnerability, pain or reassurance in response to touch, but at the same time might be so unused to the idea that their body can communicate with them at all that they just don't experience, or fail to notice, or perhaps subliminally censor the signals that are coming from body to mind. From the start, to make it easier for clients to access their own mind/body metaphors, Clean Touch encourages a 'metaphor-friendly' approach, using the proactive coaching style of Caitlin Walker's (2014, p.30) 'Clean Set-Up' questions to help the receiver to explore not just what they want from the session, but also what kind of relationship they want with themselves and with the person giving the touch. So once people have paired up into client and practitioner roles, the first three questions the practitioner asks the client are:

- *For this session to be exactly what you need,* **it will be like what?**

- **And when** *this session is like [first answer],* **you need to be like what?**

- **And** *for this session to be [first answer], and you to be [second answer],* **I need to be like what?**

Notice the '...like what?' at the end of each question, like the hook at the end of a line, fishing for metaphors. Maybe you'll get one and maybe you won't, but to get an idea of just how surprising it is to be asked these questions, let's go back to my own experience as a receiver. When my partner asks me, 'For this session to be exactly what you need, **it will be like what?**' I notice a hint of wariness inside me at the implied assumption that I should know, that I *could* know, what the session would be like, especially since I'm doing something that I've never done before, and my partner (an academic research psychologist), has cheerfully admitted to me that he has no experience in bodywork at all. But at the same time, I can't deny that a phrase has popped fully formed into my head, even though I have no idea where it came from, so shrugging and a bit bemused, I say:

- A wind blowing through a forest of pines.

And when this session is like a wind blowing through a forest of pines, you need to be like what?
- (Again, without a moment's thought, the answer just comes) The wind.

And for this session to be like the wind blowing through a forest of pines and you to be the wind, I need to be like what?

Again the answer comes so directly that I'm starting to wonder what I'm channelling:

- The source of the wind.

None of this makes any sense to me and I say so, but as we begin the hands-on work, guided by the kind of Clean questions you know very well by now:

What kind of touch...?
And is there anything else about that touch...?
And what would you like to have happen...?

I begin to realise that I am more in charge of this process than even the wildest control freak could ever hope to be in any normal kind of bodywork session. I feel I have permission to be as honest and exact as I want to be. My years of teaching shiatsu condense themselves into a few clear instructions in answer to my partner's Clean questions. Telling him how to position himself, how to relax into it and how to imagine a flow coming through his fingers into my arm, I begin to feel a quality of touch from his hands that tells me this person is very present and making a very real connection with me. And then I begin to feel a tingling in my arm – more than a tingling – a sense of something flowing through the still-aching part of my inflamed tissues, a whooshing sensation, and this whooshing feels like it's coming not from me but from him.

It's only then I remember my answers to those questions about the wind through the pines and how I would be the wind and my partner would be the source of the wind and, well…how weird is that? Where did those answers come from? How did my habitually stubborn verbal mind, wary of being asked to fabricate metaphors, somehow surrender to this other way of knowing? And how did my bodymind come up with a perfect metaphor to describe how the two of us would be working together, even though consciously I had no idea what to expect?

> In a way it seems like a contradiction of Clean principles to deliberately solicit any particular kind of response from the client, even a metaphor. Why is metaphor so important in Clean Touch?

JE: What Clean Touch allows is that greater connectivity, that greater awareness, and that's the brilliance of metaphor, that it brings those unconscious needs, wants, desires into relationship with our conscious mind. If you just go and have bodywork 'done' to you, you don't get that conscious awareness.

JK: And there's a cohesion that comes as a result of something being verbalised and brought through into the physical in that way. It's not the same if you have the somatic experience but don't verbalise it – and there's some kind of unification process that happens when you do.

JE: For example, I used to go to massage with a therapist who would talk through every muscle as he worked on it, trying to make me aware of how I was holding myself and where the tension was. It was useful, but I don't think that having someone tell you about what's going on in your body like that is as effective as generating that awareness through a process like Clean Touch, and through metaphors that you generate yourself. If you create that awareness, that is really empowering.

What about all those clients who don't spontaneously come up with a metaphor?

JE: Sometimes people haven't got to that point of working with metaphor, but if you just keep coming back to what they said they wanted to have happen at the start of the session and use that as a reference point as you work, you can just ask those two questions, 'What happens next?' and 'What's happening now?' All that can be very effective even when a client hasn't offered you any direct metaphor to work with.

JC: And you can word it in ways that make it more okay for them to access that metaphorical level of information. For example: 'I'm going to ask you some questions and these questions might sound a little strange, but if you just can say whatever comes into your head, that'll give us something to start working with.'

JE: Also, I've sometimes done a normal massage session that quite spontaneously went into metaphor and the client went with it, but afterwards they have a kind of reaction to it and think, 'What was that all about?' Clean Touch helps to get over that gap between the direct experience in the session and how the client's everyday mind makes sense of that experience afterwards.

How about when a client drifts off into a state of deep relaxation and isn't really consciously present?

JC: Those are really interesting boundaries to be exploring. When you've got this other person working with you, giving their whole attention to you, at what point does it become less than optimum that the client's just zoned out? At what point does the facilitator take responsibility to question that? Maybe you can link it back to the set-up and the intention for the session, and perhaps the last thing that they said. Or if they get to a point where they're completely gone and they don't know what's happening next, is it the facilitator's responsibility to help them move beyond that so they don't just spend an hour in that 'Don't know' place? And when is it useful for me to bring in some of my own expertise from a training system or from an intuition or something the client said previously? Where is the point to be proactive, while all the time being ready to say, 'Well actually you're telling me you want to zone out and that's okay'? Of course, you can always ask, '**And when** you'd like to zone out, **is there anything else** about zoning out?'

Impressed by the sheer variety of responses that came up during the workshop, I asked a few other participants about their experience of Clean Touch. Jane Clappison has more than 20 years' experience as a physiotherapist and has also trained in CranioSacral therapy and the Alexander technique. She knows very well how powerful the changes that may happen for people in both one-to-one sessions and in mind/body training workshops can be, so I was interested to know how Clean Touch compared to her previous experience.

What happened for you in the Clean Touch workshop?

I enjoyed where it took me, and that in such a short space of time it helped resolve something for me. I had developed some sciatic pain as I was driving home the day before, and as I let the images emerge, they seemed to connect with what had happened that day at work, so it was very immediate for me. In that exercise there were two people working on me at the same time, and the first places I asked to be touched were my hip and my eyes. I wanted my eyes covered up, and I started getting this sense of being like a bear in a cave in the dark being very grumpy, and then I realised I was feeling grumpy about something that happened at work, and then I realised that I was in a cave to get away from it all, and that resolved during the session. Not just my frustration but the sciatic pain too!

How would you compare it to other kinds of bodywork?

In some ways it felt quite similar to experiencing CranioSacral therapy, but in cranial work the practitioner is using their intuition, whereas in Clean Touch I could ask for what I wanted. In cranial we often move the person about, but in Clean Touch you have real freedom to move as you want to; you don't even have to be lying down, you can be standing up or walking around. I really enjoyed that as the receiver, and by the end of the workshop I could see that people were really thrilled with it, that something could be so powerful. Then after the workshop I tried combining Clean Touch with CranioSacral with a client I regularly see and it was really effective. I liked that she was able to take a much more active part in the process and that she could ask for the kind of touch she wanted.

Another participant, Tamsin Hartley, also enjoyed this sense of partnership between client and facilitator:

You've been a physiotherapist and now you work as a coach and have trained in Clean Language; that's an interesting background to bring to Clean Touch.

Yes, for me Clean Touch is a real combination of the skills that I feel very comfortable with. I found it a beautiful way of working with touch, very empowering and much more of an interplay than, say, having a therapeutic massage. In Clean Touch it feels much more like a partnership, and so much more respectful somehow.

And when it's so much more like a partnership, what's important about that?

Through facilitating people with Clean Language in coaching, I've come to realise that it's okay to let the other person lead. It's beautiful to let the receiver of touch take the lead and for me as the facilitator to be comfortable with that and with not knowing what's going to happen next. For example, I once had a body therapy session from someone who seemed to work very intuitively. Whilst it felt fantastic, there was something quite shocking for me about his approach because at various points he told me his intuitions about me. I felt myself wanting to put up a bit of resistance to that, like, 'Hang on a minute, what do you know about my body that I don't?' I feel that being 'Cleaner' would have avoided this reaction in me and possibly been more effective.

What happened for you personally as a receiver during the Clean Touch workshop?

As a receiver of Clean Touch you quite quickly and intensively get to the point that you need to get to as the receiver because you're in control and you're the one asking for touch and the kind of touch you want. For me, touch on certain places brought up memories and metaphors that really surprised me. There was a point at which I asked to be touched on my shoulder, and it immediately brought back, in a very safe way, memories from childhood – it was almost like those memories were locked in that place. That was fascinating. And at the same time, it felt like I was just exploring for myself, rather than someone suggesting an analysis or an explanation.

And what can you take away with you from the workshop?

There's something about being a receiver with Clean Touch that I can take with me and take forward. Because there were metaphors attached to the body sensations, if I remind myself of the metaphor it helps me to reconnect with the touch and the information I got from those sensations. For example, if I feel my shoulder tension again I can just tune in and ask myself, 'What's happening now?', and it helps me reconnect with the metaphors I experienced on that day.

And how about the relational aspects of Clean Touch?

As the receiver, when the way you want to be touched isn't the way the giver does it, there can be something to learn in that. I've had this experience, and there was a learning that I gained from accepting the touch when it wasn't quite as I thought I wanted it to be – there was an interplay to adapting to the kind of touch the giver could give.

And what was it about that adapting?

Maybe for me as the receiver there could be metaphoric information in the fact that it wasn't the touch I wanted it to be – a lack of toughness, perhaps, or a lack of strength, could then be metaphoric for other experiences where something wasn't as strong as I wanted it. So I can explore that in other situations in my life, when something isn't as I expected it to be.

And the opposite of that, the opportunity Clean Touch gives you to be assertive about the kind of touch you want?

Yes, that can be powerful too. In one exercise when I was a giver of touch, I think that just being able to ask for touch was very emotional for the other person, just to know that she could ask for something and have someone respond in that way, through touch.

How might you use Clean Touch when you're working with clients in your coaching sessions?

Normally with coaching clients, I don't say, 'Now we're going to use Clean Language'. I just follow them with Clean questions if they start to use a metaphor, so if I hadn't pre-framed that the session would involve Clean Touch, I might say, 'If you like, this is something we can explore through touch. And with touch you can be seated or standing or maybe lying on a mat, with your clothes on' and 'I would just ask if, in relation to this issue, there's a part of your body that would like to receive touch.' So it's still part of their choice, and then you have another modality of working Cleanly in a coaching session.

Back in the workshop but now as the facilitator, I'm noticing how Clean Touch makes it easy to observe direct somatic responses that arise as my partner explores a metaphor. I ask:

*And that tightness in your shoulders **is like what?***
- (His reply comes softly spoken and sounding like a question) A fossil?

*And when that tightness is like a fossil, **where would it like to be touched?***

He directs my hand to a spot between his shoulder blades and we work on getting the touch to feel just right. Soon his breathing starts to deepen.

And what's happening now?
- The fossil is relaxing from the stone.

For a moment I am lost in the pure poetry of the metaphor, wondering what a fossil would be like if it could relax from the very thing that holds its form; and wondering too at the implied timespan of how long this symptom has been a part of his body. These wonderings are all mine, of course, not necessarily my partner's, but my hand is already feeling a softening of muscles and fascia.

And when the fossil is relaxing from the stone, **then what happens?**
- Its body becomes like a jelly.

Now my partner's shoulders start to move, actively searching for the right position and the right rhythm of movement that will allow something to release.

And when its body becomes like a jelly, and moving your shoulders, **then what happens?**
- (There's a pause as the question sinks in) The jelly becomes my body.

My hand just rests there as my partner takes some time to get used to a body that feels more like a jelly than a fossil in a stone. Eventually I have the sense of a movement being complete, so I ask:

And how are you now?
- Very relaxed…(a long pause)…very in my body…very grounded.

There is a hint of a smile.

And that place between your shoulders, **how is that now?**

The smile disappears into a blank look – the sort of blank look you have when you can't find something that was there a minute ago.

- Mmm. Seems okay there now.

The blank look turns into a gentle frown, as if some sceptical part needs to be convinced that this wasn't all just some kind of game with metaphors. This is a natural part of the process for most people as they shift from their more body-connected consciousness back to the desktop of their everyday mind. Sometimes all that's needed is a moment to acknowledge that.

And is there anything else?
- No, that's fine.

The frown disappears.

And would that be a good place to finish?

The smile is back again, along with a full-bodied stretch that seems to come from somewhere very deep inside; the sort of stretch a fossil would make, perhaps, after a hundred million years in a stone.

Because Clean Touch is a process rather than a technique or a therapy, it can be applied in many ways. Perhaps at least a taste of it should be included in any kind of bodywork training, so that practitioners who are used to an expert/patient model as in acupuncture or osteopathy, or a teacher/student model as in Feldenkrais or the Alexander Technique, can have a hands-on experience of what it's like at the other end of the spectrum of relationship between therapist and client – a place where, significantly, the words to describe the two roles do not come so easily. In the Clean Language community, 'facilitator' and 'explorer' are often used to describe these roles, though 'explorer' may sound a bit too intrepidly outward-bound for some people. 'Giver' and 'receiver' are the terms that Jackie and Jeni use in their workshops, but they freely admit that they don't really do justice to the dynamics of the Clean Touch relationship.

A TRIANGLE OF AWARENESS

Clean Touch offers bodywork therapists who have no qualifications in a psychological therapy a very safe way to acknowledge and work with issues clients may have, for example about boundaries or control, especially where there has been trauma or abuse. It can also help both client and therapist recognise information that arises during bodywork from the interaction between them. For instance, in one workshop the giver was asking Clean questions about exactly what direction of touch would be right for the receiver, and not getting very clear answers. Finally the receiver said, 'It doesn't matter about the direction,' and as soon as she said it, realised that the real issue her body was trying to get her to recognise was to do with a problem about finding a sense of direction in her life. She used the rest of the session to explore that.

This example is a good illustration of how Clean Touch can both challenge and extend a bodywork practitioner's sense of what is possible. In their workshops Jackie and Jeni talk about the triangle of awareness the facilitator's attention moves through as they work with Clean Touch.

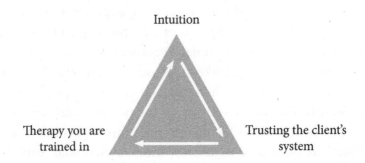

A triangle of awareness

As a practitioner, you're used to following the principles of whatever therapy you're trained in, and the more experienced you become, you also get used to following your intuitions. Clean Touch invites you into the third corner of the triangle where the client takes the lead in a deliberate and conscious way. Here, the more experienced you are as a practitioner, the more challenging this corner can be to your preconceived notions of what you should do or your intuitive sense of what you want to do. You will still find yourself picking up the usual signals about what their body is telling you and where and how you'd like to work. What you do with those signals is up to you. You can simply notice them arising, acknowledge them and let them go, or you can put them to one side to see if they connect with anything that comes up for your client later in the session (as in the case study that follows). The dynamics of the therapeutic 'field' between client and practitioner are so dense with information flowing in both directions that simply bringing that kind of mindful awareness to these signals can, in ways we can't yet fully explain in any scientific way but that we often experience, powerfully amplify sensations and intuitions that might otherwise remain out of the client's awareness.

~ 32 ~

APPROACHING CHILDBIRTH
WITH CLEAN TOUCH

A CASE STUDY

Here's an example of how I use a modified kind of Clean Touch when a woman in her mid-20s comes to see me in the last trimester of her first pregnancy. She has no experience of Clean Language and very little experience of any kind of bodywork; she just wants some help for the physical aches and pains which, as far as she can tell, are a natural part of the latter stages of her pregnancy. Though she seems willing enough to play the game as I ask her some Clean questions, each time I ask her what she'd like to have happen, her answers sooner or later snap back like an overstretched elastic to focus on her problem, the 'aches and pains'. Underneath her open and cheerful manner, she looks so tired that I wonder if the best way to help her relax into getting a genuinely felt sense of an outcome would be to ask if she'd like to lie down so that we can start to find out what those aches and pains are all about.

She's very happy to, and as I talk her through a simple mindfulness exercise I often use at the start of a session to help clients settle down and start listening to their own body, she immediately drifts off into a few minutes of light sleep – her bodymind's first answer to what *it* would like to have happen! Using this time to tune in to the signals I'm getting from her energy channels, I'm drawn more and more to her lower back. I let my attention rest there until she opens her eyes again, ready for a bit of Clean Touch.

And when you gently scan through your whole body, where would it like to be touched?

Sure enough, the first place she says that she's aware of is her lower back.

I say that this is where my attention was also being drawn to – not a very Clean thing to do, and I wouldn't say it to every client, but at this stage of the session, I feels like it would help to build a sense of trust and teamwork, not just between me and my client but between her and her own bodymind. I already know exactly where in her lower back I want to start working, but that's not the point in Clean Touch, so I ask:

And whereabouts in your lower back?

Lying on her right side, she lets her left hand feel around until it finds a particular spot in the lumbar area.

And what kind of feeling is that?
 – A pulling-in feeling.

Anything else about that pulling-in feeling?
 – As if the muscles there are weak, not strong.

And when there's a pulling-in feeling, as if the muscles there are weak, not strong, is that near the surface or deeper inside?
 – It goes in deeper, not just on the surface.

I'll put my hand on the place you pointed to, and you tell me if that's exactly the right spot, or if you want it to move a bit.

My thumb goes to a point right on the spine, and I quickly feel a response, a sense of energy starting to move and come into this point, which felt stiff and rather empty before. The client doesn't say anything, but seems quite absorbed, just feeling what's happening there. Eventually, I ask:

And what's happening now?
- Yeah, it's changing. Now it's going lower down – it wants some attention down there.

Again she gestures with her hand to her upper sacrum. When I put my hand there, the feeling is quite different – a very obvious lack of response, as if there's no resilience there, like pressing into the sole of a well-used running shoe that's lost all its bounce. And even more significantly, nothing seems to be happening there even though I'm keeping my thumb on the point patiently for some time. My own sense is that this point is saying, 'No one's going to listen to me, so I'm going to have to do this all by myself' – a common-enough refrain from parts of the body a person has for whatever reason become disconnected from. But when there's no response from the body, in my experience that's a good moment to bring the client's conscious awareness to that place, so I ask her what she's feeling there.

- Yeah, that bit feels kind of isolated from the rest of my body.

Deliberately deviating from a Clean approach, and feeling a bit like I'm talking to a couple who have drifted apart, I tell her about my sense that it's not responding because it doesn't think anyone will listen to it.

- I think I've been ignoring it, actually.

And what happens when *you just keep your attention on it there?*

Although that last question starts with '**And what happens…?**' it isn't really a Clean question; actually it's a suggestion to use a simple mindfulness technique, but putting it in the form of a question keeps some continuity with the Clean Touch format. With my hand still there, I gradually feel energy starting to flow into that area. When I ask her, so can she:

- Yeah, I feel like it's starting to be part of me again, not sectioned off.

In a nice demonstration that she's got the idea of Clean Touch even though I haven't specifically said much about it as a way of working; she then asks me to work two lines corresponding to the sacro-ileac joints, saying that's where the feeling has moved to now.

As I work these, the touch there seems to say that the whole pelvis wants to widen laterally. I don't mention this since it seems a pretty obvious thing for a pelvis to want to do in the later stages of pregnancy, but I make a mental note, holding it in my awareness as I continue to work down her legs. Now, with her pregnant belly, she has shifted to lying on her back with her knees well supported by pillows. I'm moving out of pure Clean Touch mode and simply following my hands, not asking her for directions but checking in with her for how each contact feels and if it's in exactly the right place for her.

When I come to the lateral side of her left foot I notice the same 'Nobody's listening to me' sense that I experienced on the sacrum. Somehow this one seems to have even more of a psychological edge to it. I know from meridian theory that the emotion connected with this channel is fear, and I ask myself some Clean questions silently about what I'm aware of there. Often an area I've been drawn to has something to say, and a tone it wants to say it in. But with this point on the foot, there just seems to be silence. Okay then, a good point to go back into Clean Touch mode rather than trying to be the expert who can sort things out all by myself. But what to ask? Guided partly by theory (the 'fear') and partly by what the pelvis has already told me (about wanting to widen), I empty my mind to see what kind of question pops into it:

*And the actual experience of giving birth, **what happens when** you think about that?*

Notice that, like my suggestion to try a bit of mindful focusing earlier, this appears to be a question but the last three words – '...think about that' – are what in hypnosis is called an embedded command. Not very Clean at all, except in the sense that it's the question that emerged. It's also a very obvious question, and some practitioners might have asked it a lot earlier in the session. Here it just felt that the timing was right. The combination of Clean Touch and a more intuitive approach seems to have got us to the part of her bodymind that's holding the fear. So how will she answer the question about giving birth?

- I'm curious about how it will be...(a long pause)...and it's also scary, thinking about how the muscles just take over, and that I might lose connection with the baby if things don't go properly, like if something gets stuck and the baby isn't coming out.

And where is scary?
- Umm, it's not like it's anywhere in my body, so it must be like a thought in my head.

Whereabouts in your head?
- Sort of in the middle, about level with my eyes.

And is there anything else about that thought in the middle of your head?
- I see it's just like a negative thought; it's not actually real. It's just my head going through all the possible things that might happen and getting anxious about it.

As she says this, the area I'm working on in the side of her foot responds at last, starting to feel more alive. Thinking about her last response, I realise there are two different parts to that negative thought – the part about the muscles taking over and the part about losing connection to the baby, so I decide to check them both separately.

And when it's just a negative thought about your muscles taking over, is there anything else about that?

Rather than going further into a 'felt sense' or metaphorical kind of response, she starts talking about a strategy – how she's aiming to use her breathing to stay in the moment so that she won't panic when her muscles do take over.

The other part seems very important too, so I ask:

And losing connection with the baby: **what kind of** connection with the baby **is that** connection?

I could have asked about 'losing', which might have taken us deeper into what 'scary' was all about, but I choose to go for 'connection' here and see what response it gets.

– Right now, it's harmonious and nice. I'm not feeling irritated by the baby, or anything like that.

And **when** the connection with the baby is harmonious and nice, **then what happens?**
– It feels good, like it's all relaxing down around my pelvis area.

An 'A-ha!' moment for me. Without mentioning what I'd felt before – that sense of her pelvis wanting to widen – it has somehow found its way into her conscious awareness.

And **is there anything else about** all relaxing down around your pelvis area?
– Yeah, in fact it feels good all over my body.

I can feel this relaxing too now, as I come back to check the lower back and sacral areas where we began.

We agree that's a good place to finish off, and go back over the session, comparing what we both noticed and felt, and I ask her what the main things she's got from the session are. She says the key things for her were realising that she'd been deliberately ignoring her lower back so that she could 'Get things done', and also noticing how she started to relax there during the session as she really paid attention to it. We discuss how she could take that discovery home with her, so that when she feels she has to ignore her lower back to get things done she could promise to pay some attention to it later on.

It would be nice to say that following this session the birth itself was easy. Actually it turned out to be anything but. She was in labour for three days virtually without sleep, with a baby that weighed over ten pounds. Sheer exhaustion meant that she needed an epidural to deal with the pain and an episiotomy to help the baby out. After the birth, the cord to the placenta broke and had to be removed surgically. Overall, she lost so much blood that she had to have a transfusion. What was remarkable was how quickly both mother and baby recovered from this ordeal. She told me later that she'd been confident throughout that everything would turn out well and that, after the birth, instead of dwelling on how hard it had been, she had deliberately spent time reassuring her body that it had done a good job. 'I imagined bits of me getting better,' she said, and within a few days had recovered surprisingly well from both the exhaustion and the physical trauma.

There's no way of knowing how much our session ten weeks before had helped her to develop that resilience, but for me, this session was a useful example of how someone wanting simply to deal with her 'aches and pains' can get some insight into what those aches and pains are all about and how to listen better to her body as it prepares for the huge challenge of childbirth. However you incorporate it into your work, Clean Touch is a very effective way of putting the client at the centre of the process, allowing them to be as proactive as they want to be in discovering those 'unknown knowns' that live somewhere between mind and body and which, with your help, they can access through metaphor, touch and a willingness to trust whatever emerges.

3.5 INTERVIEWS WITH PRACTITIONERS WHO USE CLEAN LANGUAGE

CLEAN LANGUAGE
AND ACUPUNCTURE

Paul Silk BA, BSc, ITEC, LicAc MBAcC, is a London-based acupuncturist who also practises sports and deep tissue massage and several Eastern and Western movement arts, including tai chi, qi gong and circus acts such as static trapeze and rope.

I love using Clean Language because acupuncture needles can create strange sensations and it really helps to have a set of tools that say, 'That's like what?' or 'Whereabouts is that?' or 'That's weird like what?' It's really useful just to be able to help clients unpack the sensations that they're having. With Clean Language, my most productive technique is simply to echo what the client has just said and let them process what it is they are feeling, and that is very helpful, for them and for me. Maybe a person doesn't want or need a metaphor landscape, but I can still use Clean questions to help them. You have to be able to hear what the client wants.

Also, it's very different from the normal way of doing acupuncture that we get from China. With this approach, clients are not just there to be passive and to be stuck to the table with needles. Their active experience of needling also becomes part of the treatment and, with Clean questions, I can really help them focus on what they're actually feeling.

For example, sometimes a client will have a metaphor for their physical sensations or their embodied feelings before I've even asked a Clean question. When they say, 'It's like this burning that travels from here to here,' it's as if they're asking if what they're feeling is real, or normal. So in many cases, it's fine to use Clean Language without telling the client what you're doing. But when you're iterating people's words and feeding that back to them, that's not normal. Sometimes you see they've noticed and you have to make a decision, 'Do I stay with this or do we just go back into conversation?' I had one client with a real sensitivity to language who just physically contorted when I started using Clean. I had to come way out of it and be utterly conversational and use humour to break the moment before I was able to go back in.

A lot of clients take time to start trusting the answers that come to them. You see their eyes moving and then they say, 'Oh no, I can't really think of anything.' I had one client who started every answer with, 'The only thing I can think of is...' That went on for two sessions, but by the third one they were comfortable with the process and didn't need to say that any more. And as we work, I'm always checking, 'Does that make sense?' Quite a lot of the feedback clients give me is, 'It felt uncomfortable but that was okay. I was able to stay uncomfortable with it.'

Obviously, I can't say if it improves the efficacy of the treatment, because you'd need a proper research study to show that, but I absolutely believe it improves rapport, and the better your rapport, the more the client can access their parasympathetic nervous system, and that's where all the healing takes place. Even if that was the only thing that Clean Language did, I'd use it just for that.

CRANIOSACRAL THERAPY

Jane Clappison MSTAT, MCSP, MCSS, is an Alexander Technique teacher, Chartered Physiotherapist and CranioSacral therapist based in East Yorkshire.

When I first heard them, Clean questions sounded very similar to the sort of questions we were trained to ask in the somato-emotional release module of my CranioSacral training: 'And what's that? And what's that about? Is that familiar?' But in somato-emotional release, the idea is to get the person to remember the trauma or event so that it can be resolved. What I found uncomfortable about that was that if I wasn't doing it well, I was re-traumatising people and not achieving a resolution of the problem. That's where Clean Language got me off the hook. With Clean I don't even have to understand what they're talking about, I just have to use the questions. Even when you get it wrong, you're just getting more information. There's less dissonance with the client, too, because I'm using their language. There's less room for misunderstanding.

I don't use the Clean approach to start a session. It's just, 'Can you lay down on your back comfortably?' and then I talk about how I do the assessment by laying my hands on in various places. So I'm already there with my hands on before I start asking Clean questions. With cranial we're looking for what we call 'energy cysts', and if I do find one and put my hands on it then it may or may not release. If it doesn't, then that's the point when I would normally start to dialogue with the person.

Normally, I say the aim is to release this energy cyst, and that talking about it usually helps it to release quicker, and would they be okay with that? I also say that I use something called Clean Language, which sounds a bit strange but would it be okay if I use that? And I've never had anybody say 'No' so far. Then I'll usually ask, 'What are you noticing?' or 'What are you sensing?' That's not one of the official Clean questions, but it's usually what I start with.

Then I'll use the basic Clean questions, for example if they say it's painful, I might ask, '**And what kind of** painful **is that** painful?'

While I'm talking with them, I'm also using the connection through my hands to see how the tissue is responding to what I do. As we go on with the Clean questions, they'll get to a point where they can say what it needs. Let's say it needs love, for example, 'And can it have love?' or 'Can you give it love?' and then, 'And can that happen now?' And I can feel the tissues release. It's quite wonderful really, that the two things work together.

With cranial work, once I'm working at an energy cyst, the language that emerges is theirs, and I follow the tissues. If it was really Clean I'd ask them what they wanted me to do next, which I don't. I have a framework that I'm working with. Somehow I can keep the two separate. Usually I'm doing very little, just hanging on. I think my metaphor for working with clients like this would be that it's a bit like holding on to the string of a kite!

CLEAN LANGUAGE
AND YOGA NIDRA

Ben Wolff is a yoga teacher, yoga teacher trainer and a clinical hypnotherapist based in London.

I got interested in Clean Language because, as a yoga teacher, I realised that the best way to communicate with people was through metaphor. I noticed, for example, that in yoga many of the poses have metaphorical names like 'tree pose' or 'warrior pose'. I'd already come across metaphor in hypnotherapy and Neuro-Linguistic Programming (NLP), so I was searching for good metaphors to use when teaching yoga, and that eventually got me to this obscure thing called Clean Language.

Compared to other therapies, I loved the fact that Clean Language took me as the therapist out of the client's experience. In the development of any therapy, the original intention is absolutely crucial to how it manifests, and I felt with David Grove that his original intention was to get completely out of the client's way and to help them help themselves.

My speciality is Yoga nidra, which is the meditative heart of yoga, the lovely bit at the end where you lie down and don't have to do anything and the teacher is talking. That's normally a monologue but I sometimes use it as a dialogue, and I use a Clean approach to do that. For instance, one of the things I do stems back to an ancient Zen technique, where we're in the space of Yoga nidra and I invite people to visit four different imaginary rooms. There's a room of Happiness, a room of Joy, a room of Harmony and a room of Bliss. As we walk through the four rooms, I'll ask Clean questions that sometimes have wordless answers. This is one of the things that is brilliant about it – you can always use the word 'That' for whatever people have got in their heads, rather than them having to say anything out loud. '**That** room of Happiness, **that's like what? Is there anything else about that?** And when you look can you see if there's a colour, a location, a size or a shape? And whereabouts are you feeling these things?' That's a Clean approach because you haven't put anything in their heads, apart from having put them in a room of Happiness.

In some ways there's not much difference between putting someone in a room of Happiness and asking them, '**And what would you like to have happen?**' The point is we're in a space of meditation, we're breathing coherently at five breaths a minute, we've got all the power of Yoga nidra, and then we add some Clean Language as well. That's a pretty powerful combination!

What happens is that people have insight, and I think Clean Language really helps to stimulate that. There's a part of the brain, the anterior superior temporal gyrus, which fMRI scans show is activated in moments of insight, and my aim is to make that fire repeatedly because, as they say, 'Neurons that fire together, wire together'. So with the help of Clean questions, we're increasingly shutting down the left hemisphere and increasingly moving to the right hemisphere, until you get to that amazing wordless space beyond metaphor and beyond language. By that point it's almost nothing to do with you as the practitioner, since client and therapist are intuitively working as one. And you can use the bridge of Clean Language to get you there. So Clean Language is now my operating system; it's how I've rewired my brain.

YOGA AND THE OUTCOME QUESTION

Rosaleen Bloomfield is a qualified Alignment-based yoga teacher, a Symbolic Modelling and Systemic Modelling facilitator, Institute of Leadership and Management coach and mentor, and founder of Yoga Blooming, based in south-west London.

When I started to learn Clean Language I thought, 'There's a lot of yoga in this,' in the sense that they're both about developing self-awareness and paying attention to the mind/body. Tensions in the body can reflect psychological tensions, and a well-timed Clean question can bring an 'A-ha!' moment about other things going on in a person's life.

When I use Clean in a yoga class, first I get people to come up with an outcome – when you do that you can see them behaving very differently in the class. For example, an outcome may be 'I want to let go of anger' or 'I want to have mental clarity'. Then I ask, '**And what needs to happen** for you to get that?' Then they lie on the floor and do basic relaxation with Clean questions. If I'm doing a yoga breathing session, I'll ask them to focus specifically on breath awareness with Clean questions adapted for breathing, like, 'What's between the end of the outbreath and the beginning of the inbreath?' Then at the end we come back to the outcomes and how they are now.

Using this kind of language helps to keep each person's experience Clean. Instead of saying, 'Your breathing is much deeper now,' I'll ask, '**And** now your breathing **is like what?**' That can work really well. For example, one person had a real issue with breathing and came up with a metaphor about being out in a boat and the sea being very calm, and she finds the metaphor works for her now whenever she needs to calm her breathing down.

Another example would be in a chakra workshop. I remind myself that I have no idea what each participant understands by the word 'energy', so I'll ask Caitlin Walker's metaphor elicitation question: 'When your energy is at its best, **it's like what?**' (Walker 2014, p.72). And then I ask the whole group Clean questions so they can discover more about what came up for them, for example, '**What kind of** energy? **And is there anything else about** that energy? **And where is** that energy?'

And then I'll ask them to draw their own metaphor and to pair up and ask each person to tell their partner about their metaphor. It works really well because then they realise that each other's ideas about energy can be very different. It creates more understanding in the group of each person's way of seeing and being in the world, and allows them to connect and interact with one another at a different level. So throughout the workshop I get them to come back to their personal metaphor, noticing how they can embody that metaphor now.

I also use Clean when I'm doing yoga one to one, for example to facilitate a back problem. I ask the client to create a metaphor for the pain so they can discover more about it…what it's like, as well as where it is, what size or shape it has, and so on. Then I have a clearer idea of what yoga posture we can use, and I use Clean questions to check what they're experiencing and direct their attention more deeply. In the end, it's all about allowing the client to go deeper into their own stuff, and I find that Clean is a good way to do that.

PHYSIOTHERAPY WITH
CLEAN LANGUAGE

Sioelan Tjoa BSc, MSc (Exercise Physiology), MCSP, MACP, AACP, HPC, certified NLP practitioner (INLPTA), works as a private physiotherapy practitioner in Cumbria and has worked for many years in the UK National Health Service as a clinical specialist.

I always thought that to be the best I could be I just needed more knowledge of medical and technical skills. It wasn't until I did an NHS in-house coaching course and then discovered Clean Language that I started to realise it's the client who's the specialist, not me. I'm providing them with firm technical support and at the same time nurturing their ability to help themselves.

Traditionally in physiotherapy you ask about quality, severity and location of pain and about what might ease symptoms. You also ask about the history and mechanics of an injury. You try to narrow it down to the anatomical structure and pain mechanisms and what underlying structure is at fault. All of this externalises the client's problem, and sets up the expectation that the physiotherapist, being the specialist, will find the answer.

Patients aren't used to being asked about what resources they have. They may be relying on advice and beliefs from their doctor or other health professionals and can seem quite disempowered. During my coaching course I got the insight that the type of information and advice a patient needs depends on their levels of knowledge, motivation and willingness to change.

If I ask Clean questions, it changes the client's perspective from 'You're the expert' to helping them focus on their own issues and explore their own solutions. Potentially, it makes them start to realise that they are the expert, and maybe then they can start to see me as a facilitator in their process of healing instead of the specialist who's going to fix them.

If I'm integrating Clean questions with normal questions, some people get a bit suspicious and look at me with an expression that says, 'Where are you going with this?' Or you ask what they want and they say, 'I want the pain to go away.' Some people do shut down. With other people it just flows, and I'm starting to use Clean Language now without thinking about it, and it's incredibly powerful in getting to the essence of people's issues. Then things just emerge as you go along, which is fascinating.

I had a very interesting guy with cancer, with massive scars from his operation and a protruding hernia there. But the problem he came with was leg pain, which was stopping him from walking any distance. The point for him was that he really enjoyed walking. In my head I was thinking, what could it be? Spinal referred to the leg? A circulatory problem? A mechanical problem from the fact that he doesn't have a normal abdominal musculature any more? But I was asking Clean questions right from the start, so the patient very much felt I was listening to him to find out what he wanted to have happen. It turned out that it wasn't the pain that was the main problem for him; it was the restricted range of movement that the pain was causing. But you could have easily homed into the pain, and missed the fact that it was really about his mobility.

I gave him some exercises and he asked, 'How often should I be doing this?' So I asked, 'How often could you be doing it?' and he said, 'Every hour'. I asked if he wanted to do it that often, and he said, 'Yes, if it makes me better.' So rather than giving the patient a sheet of exercises to do, and being very prescriptive, it's like asking, 'What would you like to do?', and then asking, 'What do you feel able to do?'

In the NHS you see people for all kinds of reasons, whether they're motivated to help themselves or not. Patients don't expect to be asked what it is they want. Their doctor might have given them a prescription – 'Here are your tablets, here is your cream, go and see the physio' – and it's all a confirmation that the pain is really genuine; but no one has really asked, '**What would you like to have happen?**'

TEACHING TAI CHI WITH CLEAN QUESTIONS

Helen Holden is an experienced tai chi instructor and shiatsu therapist, based near Plymouth in the UK.

I run a class for older people and I find the students are only too happy to come in and discuss all their joint problems with me before we get started – hip replacements, aching knees and so on. This particular lady was new to the class and she greeted me with an angry tirade about all her health issues and about not being listened to by her doctor. Her main problem was a slow recovery from hip replacement surgery. She was concerned about the fact that her body had become stiff through lack of exercise. I assured her she was in the right place and that she could work gently and at her own pace. Then I thought of trying some Clean questions. I asked, 'How would you like to feel after the class?' And to my surprise, even though she'd been feeling so angry about it, she immediately answered in the positive.

'I'd like to be able to move more freely and feel more balanced and relaxed.' She put her hand behind her hips at this point, naturally opening out her chest, which was previously collapsed.

'Okay, **and what would that be like**, to be able to move more freely?'

She looked a little taken aback, thought for a moment and then said, 'Like a young tree that bends and flexes in the wind. At the moment I feel like a dead old tree, all brittle and stiff.' As she told me this she opened her hands out to the side of her body, moving her hips from side to side. She was visibly connecting with her body, and as we started the class, her face was more relaxed and positive.

At the end, I managed to have a brief chat with her. Before I had a chance to ask, she said, 'I feel so much better. I was a bit stiff and creaky at first but I soon got into the flow of it.'

'And how did that feel, to get into the flow of it?'

'I felt a bit inhibited when we started, but then I really got into the movement and about halfway through the class I suddenly realised I'd forgotten all about my problems.'

I was impressed at how easily the Clean questions helped me to direct the student's attention away from her health problems and onto what she hoped to get from the session, and how easily they allowed her to connect with her body in a more positive way.

HOMEOPATHY AND
CLEAN LANGUAGE

Dr Joseph Kellerstein DC, ND, FCAH, CCH, is a chiropractor, naturopath and homeopath in Toronto, Canada, and teaches postgraduate courses at the Toronto School of Homeopathic Medicine, the Canadian School of Naturopathic Medicine and internationally.

Not long after I started out in homeopathy, I got a slew of patients with depression, and all I could get from them was 'I'm depressed.' So I went back to my teacher, a wonderful teacher, and he said, 'Joe, ask this question: "When you say depression, what do you mean?"' It was the first time I'd heard that – getting rich information to characterise a disease state.

Then I studied NLP for a number of years in the context of case-taking, and the lady I'd been studying with said, 'You know, Joe, if I was young and just starting out, I'd study Clean Language.' She had just been to Rhinebeck, New York, and seen James Lawley and Penny Tompkins, the authors of *Metaphors in Mind* (2000) and she was very impressed. So it took a few years but thanks to Wendy Sullivan, co-author of *Clean Language* (Sullivan and Rees 2008), and her online course, I started to learn.

When I use Clean Language I don't do a lot of development into metaphors. The initial interview with a patient is about two hours. We go through each syndrome and all the sensations associated with them, and what makes every condition worse and how complaints interact with other complaints. Then after I've gone through everything, what I'll do is ask, '**And when** all of this, **what would you like to have happen?**' After two hours! And I try to find out what would really be different about life. And often they'll give me stunning information that they haven't given me yet, even though I've been asking all the other questions.

One thing I've found is that patients aren't very associated to their discomforts. So I'm using Clean questions to help them get very clear with the pain, where it is, what affects it. And the most wonderful thing so far – I know it sounds trivial, but it's really helped me get far greater 'granularity' to the patient's syndromes – has been the idea of following the patient's energy and asking, '**And is there anything else about** all that?' So I'll listen for the tonal emphasis as they describe their situation. For example, I'll say, 'Tell me about a day with your rheumatoid arthritis,' and I'll carefully go through the day and I'll listen for the point at which they put the tonal emphasis in what they're describing; and I'll repeat back to them the bits that they really emphasised, and say, '**And when** all of that, **is there anything else about all that?**' And I get a far better description.

Clean language demands a real care and thoughtfulness for every word and gesture, and the ethic of not intruding with your own paradigms. And it all just sounds so simple, but it isn't: it's an incredible skill-set. There are a few who say 'What do you mean by that question?' and to those I say, 'Just play with me.' But most of them are just fine with it and most of them don't seem to notice the shift when I start using Clean syntax – they're good with it.

CLEAN LANGUAGE,
FELDENKRAIS AND MUSIC

Emily Walker is a freelance cellist based in Scotland, playing in orchestras and quartets. She is qualified in both Clean Language and the Feldenkrais method. Here she talks about how Clean Language and Feldenkrais help her bring a more mindful, embodied approach to her work as a teacher and a performer. Notice how, as she explores these connections, music becomes a metaphor for many of the ways that we connect with ourselves and our clients in mind/body therapy.

One thing I've learned from both Clean Language and Feldenkrais is that everything depends on where and how you direct your attention. Teaching music can be very tiring, but I realised that what's really tiring is when it becomes routine. Because I'm paying a different kind of attention now, the lessons become a lot more fun and the students respond really well to that.

The difference it makes is in my ability to stand back, to step aside. It's like creating a space for my students to make connections in their own time. As a music teacher, I do have to provide them with information so they can learn, but Clean stops me from marching on with my own agenda. So I 'see' them more, and I use a lighter touch. I think also there's a quality to the lessons that invites them to be more self-aware. For example, if they make a mistake I can ask, '**What just happened?**' or '**What happened just before that?**' It slows down time for them so they can get curious about the process of making that mistake, and it helps them become more interested in themselves.

One example was with a girl learning the piano. Every time she got to this passage, she'd stop and get angry with herself. I'd sit there and say nothing, and she went back to the beginning and did exactly the same thing again. After she'd done it three times, I said, 'Ah, **so what happens** just before you stop?'

'I go blank!'

'**So what happens** just before you go blank?'

'The notes just swim.'

'**And when** you go blank and the notes just swim, **what happens just before that?**'

'I just can't play the notes; I know I can't do it.'

So then I ask, '**And when** you go blank and the notes just swim, **what would you like to have happen?**'

'I'd like the notes to stay still.'

'**And what needs to happen** for the notes to stay still?'

'I need to go slower.'

Instead of me taking control and saying, 'Stop, slow down and try it again,' she came up with the solution herself. So these little questions can help her to be more aware of what she's doing and to take responsibility for it, and to stop trying so hard.

Another example was with a very talented student who not only played the piano and the cello but was also a singer. One day I asked him, '**What would you like to have happen** today?' and he said, 'I've noticed that when I play the piano it feels easy and I have a sense of flowing, but it's not like that when I play the cello. With the cello I just feel really blocked and I can't play how I want to.' It turned out that he was brought up in Ukraine and had a very strict Russian cello teacher, so his past with the cello had been extremely regimented. Using Clean questions, I asked, '**And when** you feel really blocked and you can't play how you want to, **what would you like to have happen?**', and he said, 'I'd like to play the cello with the same ease that I play the piano.'

So I got him to play something on the piano and asked, '**When** you're playing like that on the piano, and it's flowing, **that's like what?**' He started describing it and gesturing with his hands how it felt for him – it was really beautiful – and I said, 'Okay, now come to your cello, and play something,' and he did, and I asked him, '**That's like what?**' and he said, 'Oh, my throat gets blocked and my arms become tight.' So I said, 'Go back to the piano; what's happening in your arms when you're playing the piano?' and so on, and we started transferring his piano skills to the cello. Then at the end of the lesson he had a sort of 'A-ha!' where he realised what he *really* wanted to do – to compose a piece for cello, piano and voice, and record himself doing all three. He's a very creative person, and he ended up composing it as his project for the whole term, and it all came out of that first Clean question: '**What would you like to have happen** today?'

MUSIC IS ABOUT THE BODY

I often get students to pay attention to their body. They always like that! As they play, I'll point to one foot and then the other foot and then to a knee, bringing their awareness into their body, because the way classical music is taught is so cerebral, so intellectual. But music is about the body, about connections and feelings, and it's often very limited in the way that it's taught. There's this idea of a really strict teacher telling you you're wrong, so I like to get them to really come into their bodies.

It's about just being really present with the sound you're making. To be really present there's a kind of accepting and listening. If someone makes a noise that doesn't please them, there's a kind of rejection, a turning away from it, but actually it's only through that feedback that you can arrive at a more beautiful sound. That mindfulness really links Clean and Feldenkrais for me – not ignoring the ugliness, not judging the ugliness. It's really important for the teacher to create that space.

THE PART TO THE WHOLE

To play in a string quartet, that's the ultimate for me. When you've got the responsibility of your part to that whole, it feels like that's a way of being present and loving and sharing, and it can be really exciting. I think that's another connection with Feldenkrais and Clean Language: In Clean it's about how do the different metaphors relate to each other in that person's interior landscape? In Feldenkrais it's about how do the different bones and muscles and tissues fit together – how do they synchronise to serve the whole body? And in an orchestra it's about how do the musicians work together to serve the music, the composer and the audience?

MUSIC AND HEALING

One more thing that's related to music, and related to touching, and related to Clean: My cello teacher, Robert Cohen, a really fantastic cellist, talks about the power of music being really healing, and as a performer, being a channel. There's something about being a channel that's very much to do with Clean, because you have to not get in the way. Of course you have to engage with the music, and know it personally, and think about it, but when you perform it you just have to let go and let it come through. When you're playing or when you're touching someone, you're really listening but you have to get out of the way and just allow that sense of letting-go and being part of a greater whole. The music might be the saddest music in the world, and it might have been written three hundred years ago, but to bring it to life in that moment – that's an amazing feeling.

3.6 A FINAL WORD

A hundred years ago, whatever the therapy and in whatever part of the world it was practised – shamanism in Siberia, acupuncture in China, psychoanalysis in Vienna – the therapeutic relationship was emphatically hierarchical, and the therapist was seen as an expert at reading what the naïve patient could know nothing of. In the past 50 years that has changed enormously. Not that it is wrong to know more than your client about a subject you have studied for many years and which they have come to you specifically for help with; rather that in various kinds of therapy it is now being recognised that allowing clients to make their own discoveries and their own connections about what is going on inside them may perhaps bring something to the process of self-healing that any amount of 'expert' help cannot. But we study hard, and derive income, status and self-esteem from having this expertise, and so it is still an extraordinarily tempting default position for any therapist to fall back into. No matter how skilled we may be at bringing simple human presence to our encounters with clients, there will always be a side of us that is only too willing – whatever questions we're asking – to disregard any answers which don't fit into our therapeutic maps. Clean Language, on the other hand, is constantly nudging us to de-emphasise what we think we know, or where we think the process should be going, or what the client should be saying, or even who we think we are.

You start out learning Clean Language as a way of getting better answers from your clients. At first it looks like a simple matter of learning a dozen or so questions which, as long as you're prepared for the different kinds of answer they produce, will help your clients interact in a different way with their own bodies – from experiencing the body as something 'other' than the mind, to learning how to engage in genuine mind/body dialogue.

But there is something else going on too. The more you learn how to ask Clean questions, the more you are learning to think in this different way. You begin to realise that Clean Language is not just another useful technique to add to your therapeutic toolkit, nor is it simply the process that develops between you and your client as you ask these peculiar questions and learn how to respond to the even more peculiar answers they elicit. No, for the therapist who takes Clean Language to heart – who is willing to embody it in the way that you have to embody any language to speak it fluently – it becomes more like a *practice*, in the same way that learning to meditate or learning yoga or qi gong are a practice; they offer us a different way of paying attention to the world and our own sense of being in it, and a profoundly different way of being with a client. The way you work with words becomes a natural prelude to the way you work with touch, and involves all the things you do through movement or touch: holding, supporting, listening, focusing, opening, questioning, inviting, connecting.

The French philosopher Louis Lavelle said, 'True love is a pure attention to the existence of the other,'[1] and in that word 'pure' there is an important hint, for me at least, about what the 'Clean'

---

1   Lavelle, L. (1939) *L'Erreur de Narcisse*, Grasset, Paris, chapter 9, section 7. Thanks to Iain McGilchrist for this reference.

in Clean Language is really about. When you begin to use it not only as a technique but as a practice, you realise just how much it demands from us as practitioners – as it should, since the questions themselves demand so much from our clients. Like other kinds of meditative practice, it gradually eats away at the left hemisphere's sense of self-importance and, through that, at our own culturally constructed sense of the importance of the self.

Clean Language becomes a form of mindfulness that we practise every time we open our mouths to ask a new question, and because the questions are so simple, once learned, you find yourself using far less mental energy to support your own side of the dialogue. Far more becomes available for attending not just to your client's words but to every other kind of communication which is there in the two bodyminds that are present in the 'betweenness' of the therapeutic field. In this way, we can both expand the limits of mind/body therapy (and at the same time know better where those limits are), while helping our clients to go beyond theirs. And the more we explore that, of course, the more we taste the exhilarating sense that words can only take us so far, even words like 'infinite' or 'wisdom' or 'love'; and that what lies beyond the words brings us freshly back – 'Just Like Starting Over', as John Lennon called the last song he ever wrote – back with a beginner's mind to the wonder of this wordless world of embodiment, movement and touch.

REFERENCES

Bateson, G. (1972) *Steps to an Ecology of Mind: collected essays in anthropology, psychiatry, evolution and epistemology*, Chicago, IL, University of Chicago Press.

Bresson, R. (1977) *Notes on Cinematography*, trans. J. Griffin, New York, Urizen.

Cooper, L. and Castellino, M. (2012) *The Five-Minute Coach*, Bancyfelin, Carmarthen, Crown House Publishing.

Cornell, A.W. (1996) *The Power of Focusing*. Oakland, CA, New Harbinger.

Cornell, A.W. (2005) *The Radical Acceptance of Everything*, Berkeley, CA, Calluna Press.

Cornell, A.W. (2013) *Focusing in Clinical Practice: the essence of change*, New York, Norton.

den Dekker, P. (2010) *The Dynamics of Standing Still: the ancient art of recharging your batteries*, Haarlem, Back2Base Publishing.

Erdman, D.V. (ed.) (2008) *The Complete Poetry and Prose of William Blake*, Berkeley, University of California Press.

Gendlin, E.T. (1978) *Focusing*, New York, Bantam Books.

Gendlin, E. (1990) 'The Small Steps of the Therapy Process: How They Come and How to Help Them Come.' In G. Lietaer, J. Rombauts and R. van Balen (eds) *Client-Centered and Experiential Psychotherapy in the Nineties*, Belgium, Leuven University Press.

Gormley, A. (2011) 'Foreword.' In E. Barnes, J. Anderson and E. Shackleton, *The Art of Medicine: over 2000 years of medicine in our lives*, Lewes, Ilex Press.

Grove, D. (2010) *History of David Grove's Work 1980–2004*, compiled by J. Mote. Available at www.cleanlanguage.co.uk/articles/articles/279/1/David-Grove-history-of-work-1980-2004/Page1.html, accessed on 25 August 2016.

Grove, D. and Panzer, B. (1989) *Resolving Traumatic Memories: metaphors and symbols in psychotherapy*, New York, Irvington.

Harland, P. (2012) *Trust Me, I'm the Patient*, London, Wayfinder Press.

Hurley, S.L. (1998) *Consciousness in Action*, Cambridge, MA and London, Harvard University Press.

Itin, P. (2007) *Shiatsu als Therapie*, Norderstedt, Satz, Umschlagdesign, Herstellung und Verlag, Books on Demand.

Kaptchuk, T.J. (1983) *Chinese Medicine: the web that has no weaver*, London, Rider.

Keller, H. (1909/2009) *The World I Live In*, New York, Cosimo.

Kishi, A. and Whieldon, A. (2011) *Sei-Ki, Life in Resonance*, London, Jessica Kingsley Publications.

Korbei, L. (2007) *Eugene Gendlin*, trans. E. Zinchitz, unpublished manuscript. (Original work published 1994.)

Lakoff, G. and Johnson, M. (1999) *Philosophy in the Flesh: the embodied mind and its challenge to western thought*, New York, Basic Books.

Larkin, P. (2003) *Collected Poems*, Victoria, Australia, The Marvell Press and London, Faber and Faber.

Lawley, J. and Tompkins, P. (2000) *Metaphors in Mind: transformation through symbolic modelling*, London, The Developing Company Press.

Levine, P.A. (1997) *Waking the Tiger: healing trauma through the body*, Berkeley, CA, North Atlantic Books.

Levine, P. (2010) *In an Unspoken Voice: how the body releases trauma and restores goodness*, Berkeley, CA, North Atlantic Books.

Linden, D.J. (2015) *Touch: the science of hand, heart and mind*, London and New York, Viking.

Masunaga, S. and Ohashi, W. (1977) *Zen Shiatsu: how to harmonize Yin and Yang for better health*, Tokyo, Japan Publications.

McGilchrist, I. (2010) *The Master and his Emissary: the divided brain and the making of the Western World*, New Haven, CT and London, Yale University Press.

Ogden, P. and Fisher, J. (2015) *Sensorimotor Psychotherapy: interventions for trauma and attachment*, New York and London, Norton.

Palmer, B. (1995) 'The development of energy.' *Journal of Shiatsu and Oriental Body Therapy*, 3, 15.

Parks, T. (2010) *Teach Us to Sit Still: a sceptic's search for health and healing*, London, Harvill Secker.

Pinker, S. (1994) *The Language Instinct*, New York, Harper Perennial Modern Classics.

Porges, S.W. (2011) *The Polyvagal Theory: neurophysiological foundations of emotions, attachment, communication and self-regulation*, New York and London, Norton.

Rothschild, B. (2000) *The Body Remembers: the psychophysiology of trauma and trauma treatment*, New York, Norton.

Rowson, J. and McGilchrist, I. (2013) *Divided Brain, Divided World: why the best part of us struggles to be heard*. Available at www.thersa.org/discover/publications-and-articles/reports/divided-brain-divided-world p.22, accessed on 22 August 2016.

Schore, A. (2010) 'The Right Brain Implicit Self: A Central Mechanism of the Psychotherapy Change Process.' In J. Petrucelli (ed.) *Knowing, Not-Knowing and Sort-of Knowing: psychoanalysis and the experience of uncertainty*, London, Karnak Books.

Siegel, D.J. (2010) *Mindsight: transform your brain with the new science of kindness*, Banbury, Oxford, One World Publications.

Sullivan, W. and Rees, J. (2008) *Clean Language: revealing metaphors and opening minds*, Bancyfelin, Camarthen, Crown House Publishing.

Taylor, J.B. (2008a) *Jill Bolte Taylor's Stroke of Insight*. TED Talk. Available at www.youtube.com/watch?v=UyyjU8fzEYU, accessed on 23 August 2016.

Taylor, J.B. (2008b) *My Stroke of Insight*, London, Hodder and Stoughton.

Tompkins, P. and Lawley, J. (2003) 'Polished Verse, Interview by John Soderlund.' *New Therapist*, South Africa, Issue 26, July/August. Available at www.cleanlanguage.co.uk/articles/articles/25/1/Polished-Verse---An-interview-with-Penny-Tompkins-and-James-Lawley/Page1.html, accessed on 25 August 2016.

Travers, P.L. (1934/1998) *Mary Poppins*, London, Collins.

van der Kolk, B. (2014) *The Body Keeps the Score: mind, brain and body in the transformation of trauma*, London, Allen Lane.

Varela, F., Thompson, E. and Rosch, E. (1991) *The Embodied Mind: cognitive science and human experience*, Cambridge, MA, MIT Press.

Walker, C. (2014) *From Contempt to Curiosity: creating the conditions for groups to collaborate*, Portchester, Fareham, Clean Publishing.

Way, M. (2013) *Clean Approaches for Coaches: how to create the conditions for change using Clean Language and Symbolic Modelling*, Portchester, Fareham, Clean Publishing.

Woolf, V. (1929/1998) *A Room of One's Own*, ed. M. Sciach, London, Hogarth Press.

Woolf, V. (2002) *On Being Ill*, Ashford, MA, Paris Press.

INDEX

Nick Pole, MA, MRSS(T) has over 25 years' experience integrating Eastern and Western approaches as a mind/body therapist. With a background in Shiatsu, NLP and Clean Language, he has also trained in Mindfulness-Based Cognitive Therapy and is the Director of London Mindful Practitioners, a group for health professionals who use mindfulness in their work. He has taught his course on Clean Language for Shiatsu therapists for over ten years in six European countries. For more details visit nickpole.com.